The Vanishing Physician-Scientist?

A VOLUME IN THE SERIES

The Culture and Politics of Health Care Work

edited by Suzanne Gordon *and* Sioban Nelson

A list of titles in this series is available at www.cornellpress.cornell.edu.

The Vanishing Physician-Scientist?

Edited by

Andrew I. Schafer, MD

ILR PRESS
an imprint of
Cornell University Press ITHACA AND LONDON

First published 2009 by Cornell University Press

Printed in the United States of America

Library of Congress Cataloging-in-Publication Data

The vanishing physician-scientist? / edited by Andrew I. Schafer.
    p. cm. — (The culture and politics of health care work)
    Includes bibliographical references and index.
    ISBN 978-0-8014-4845-4 (cloth : alk. paper)
  1. Medicine—Research.   2. Physicians.   3. Medical scientists.
I. Schafer, Andrew I.   II. Series: Culture and politics of health care work.

    R850.V36   2009
    610.72—dc22   2009019282

Cornell University Press strives to use environmentally responsible suppliers and materials to the fullest extent possible in the publishing of its books. Such materials include vegetable-based, low-VOC inks and acid-free papers that are recycled, totally chlorine-free, or partly composed of nonwood fibers. For further information, visit our website at www.cornellpress.cornell.edu.

Cloth printing   10 9 8 7 6 5 4 3 2 1

For my wife, Pauline,
and my children,
Eric, Pam, and Kate

Contents

Preface

The thesis of this book is grounded in the basic assumption that physicians have played a vital role in advancing medical knowledge throughout history, and that their participation in the medical research enterprise in the future will be if anything even more vital. Yet in the years since James Wyngaarden referred to physician-scientists as an "endangered species," the general perception has been that their situation has continued to become increasingly unstable and that they may indeed be vanishing. The position of physicians as scientists is imperiled by economic, social, cultural, and even political forces. In many ways, as the book will argue, these threats are not much different from those faced by the revered physician-scientists of previous eras. They have, however, become more complex in an increasingly complex world.

In this light, I believe that the viability and vitality of physicians as scientists in the future structure of medical research now warrants comprehensive scholarly analysis. This book is intended to distill the collective knowledge and wisdom of a remarkable group of physician-scientists and leaders of academic medicine who have approached the issue from different perspectives. All those who were invited to contribute accepted the challenge with vigor. My own job, to try to tie it all together, was a relatively simple labor of love.

There are many to whom I owe a debt of gratitude. The book was stimulated by an initiative I have been privileged to lead on behalf of the Association of Professors of Medicine. At the APM I particularly thank Charlie

Clayton, Allison Haupt, and Jessica O'Hara for their indefatigable energy and dedication to the project. The APM-sponsored first national consensus conference, "Revitalizing the Nation's Physician-Scientist Workforce," in November 2007, which I chaired, catalyzed the production of this book. It was funded through an R13 grant from the National Institutes of Health, to which, remarkably, twelve of its institutes and the Office of the Director contributed support. The initiative was also generously supported by the Burroughs Wellcome Fund; the Doris Duke Charitable Foundation; the American Academy of Allergy, Asthma, and Immunology; American Gastroenterological Association; American Society of Clinical Oncology; and American Society of Nephrology. In particular the Robert Wood Johnson Foundation provided a grant which made this publication possible.

Suzanne Gordon's outstanding editorial work as series editor has been simply invaluable. I am likewise grateful to Fran Benson at Cornell University Press for her unwavering support of this project. In my office, Beverly Borg and Silva Sergenian provided the kind of inexhaustible, expert, and meticulous preparation of the manuscript to which I have become accustomed as a very spoiled chairman of medicine. Ultimately this book would not have been produced without the lifelong inspiration of the great physician-scientists who were my own mentors: Frank Gardner, Bob Handin, William Castle, Frank Bunn, and Bill Moloney, as well as many other career role models, some of whom are themselves contributors to this book. Last but certainly not least, I wish to acknowledge the astonishing forbearance of my wife, Pauline, who has been my muse and best friend.

The Vanishing Physician-Scientist?

Introduction

Andrew I. Schafer, MD

Few members of the general public are even aware that much of the original research which has driven progress in medical knowledge throughout history has been conducted by physicians who are themselves directly involved in the practice of medicine.

Yet throughout history physicians have played a central role in advancing the science of medicine. They have brought to medical research the unique perspective of being able to ask questions inspired by their personal experience of caring for patients. Indeed, during the first half of the twentieth century, the physician's position as a "translator" of medical research predominantly took the route of pursuing clinical observations to the laboratory to elucidate mechanisms of disease, a direction referred to as "bedside-to-bench" research. With the explosive and spectacular advances in basic biomedical sciences over recent decades, the pace of which has outstripped that of clinical observation, the translator role of physicians has increasingly shifted in the opposite direction, to so-called "bench-to-bedside" research. Here the physician plays the pivotal role of applying the findings of basic science to patient care. The very essence of "translational research" is a bidirectional path between the patient and the laboratory. Thus, in order to conduct high-impact translational research, investigators throughout history have had to be able to straddle the arenas of clinical practice and basic research.

As described in detail in other chapters, concerns have been growing over the past several decades that the physician as scientist is vanishing.

In a 1979 paper in the *New England Journal of Medicine,* James Wyngaarden, who subsequently became director of the National Institutes of Health (NIH), warned that physicians who specialized in research were "an endangered species." Indeed the prospect of physicians becoming completely detached from the medical research enterprise should be of serious concern. Prior to the great rise of science in medicine during the second half of the nineteenth century, most major breakthroughs in medicine were made by doctors who devoted the majority of their time to clinical work to earn a living. Their contributions were based largely on astute observations of their patients, sometimes complemented by experiments to study them performed in what precious little time they could get away from their practices. The evolution of European university-based medical schools and dedicated research institutions, most prominently in Germany, enabled medical scientists to devote most of their effort to research and largely divorce themselves from the daily demands of patient care. All but a few of the great investigators of the late nineteenth century had medical degrees and understood the clinical relevance of their research even though they themselves were no longer much involved in the practice of medicine. A notable exception was Louis Pasteur, who was not a physician. His background was in chemistry and physics. Yet even this most famous of medical scientists in his time found his lack of formal medical training a frustrating obstacle in applying the rabies vaccine he developed to human beings.

The reform of medical education in Europe and America in the early twentieth century brought with it the integration of a rigorous scientific curriculum for physicians in training. The emergence of the individual clinical investigator that is so familiar to our generation, well educated in both clinical and scientific medicine, was fueled later in the twentieth century by the enormous growth of support for medical research by governmental agencies and philanthropies.

Now, in a world of increasingly complex clinical practice and breathtakingly rapid advances in biomedical knowledge, alternative models of medical research must again be considered. Nevertheless, the pivotal and indispensable role of physicians in the medical research enterprise is unlikely to diminish in the foreseeable future.

In this book we examine the evolution of the role of physicians as scientists ("physician-scientists") from historical, sociological, and economic perspectives. Important thought leaders in this area address current and future challenges to physicians participating in the medical research enterprise. They address the following questions: Why should it matter whether or not physicians actually engage in scientific research? How can physicians, who are trained primarily in the practice of clinical medicine, make meaningful contributions to medical research? And especially now, in the new era of genomic and molecular medicine, why should physicians even be involved in the biomedical research enterprise, which is already well populated with dedicated, full-time, "serious" scientists?

To explore these and related questions, a series of chapters discuss past, current, and future directions in the development of physician investigators, as well as their roles in academic institutions and their relationships with other types of scientists. Several chapters address the reasons for concern about the future vitality and even viability of physician-scientist careers, with particular focus on the emergence of women physicians conducting research and the impact of generational changes in the attitudes and priorities of medical school graduates. Finally, we present recent organizational initiatives to reinvigorate the clinical investigator career path.

Today the term "physician-scientist" is broadly defined as a physician (with an MD degree or an MD combined with other advanced degrees) who devotes much of his or her career to seeking new knowledge about health and disease through research. The nature of this investigative work can occupy a position anywhere along the broad continuum of biomedical research, ranging from basic science studies in the laboratory to so-called "translational" and patient-oriented clinical research, even extending to its application to the health of the population. The balance of professional effort that physician-scientists devote to research and direct patient care can vary greatly not only between individuals but also at different stages of one's career. The most productive and best-supported periods of research do indeed tend to occur when one's attention is devoted largely (and sometimes exclusively) to investigative work rather than clinical responsibilities. But this apparent correlation does not establish a clear cause-and-effect relationship. For example, a physician-scientist who is provided with ample "protected time" for research by his or her institution is probably more likely to produce creative, high-impact work than a colleague who is overwhelmed by clinical responsibilities for prolonged periods of time. Conversely, a clinically busy but insightful and motivated physician-scientist can initiate an important and novel line of research that will become well funded and will inevitably consume increasing amounts of his or her effort at the expense of time spent in patient care. The maturation of team research, as described later in this chapter, should provide further flexibility in the time commitment to research over the course of a physician-scientist's career.

Physicians have been and continue to be vital links in the medical research enterprise. Physician-scientists are in an irreplaceable and pivotal position to communicate effectively and collaborate with PhD basic scientists at one end of the medical research spectrum and with practicing health care providers at the other end.

The origins of the physician as a scientist might be traced to the very etymology of the word, which is derived from the ancient Greek *physis*, meaning "nature." In this light it is interesting to reflect on a presidential address delivered in 1888 to the British Medical Association by William Tennant Gairdner, professor of medicine at the University of Glasgow, which was titled "The Physician as Naturalist." Gairdner argued that physicians are indeed "students of nature...through personal observation." But he was not referring to them disparagingly as just the shallow, stereotypical "observing physicians" who had been so disdained by Claude Bernard earlier in the nineteenth century. He was referring to their observation of nature as merely the first step in the experimental mind of a scientific physician. In fact, in the same lecture Gairdner made the prescient comment, "I am persuaded that in a very few years the physical laboratory will become an absolutely essential preliminary step in the education of the physician of the future, and that those who have not undergone this training will be hopelessly distanced in the race." It is only as "naturalists," students of nature, that physicians can seek to be emancipated from the "mere tradition and ecclesiastical authority" of medical practice and replace it with "the spirit of modern scientific freedom...and research" (Gairdner 1889).

The Endangered Physician-Scientist

The sounding of the alarm by Wyngaarden in 1979 was based on the observation that the number of MD applicants for research grants from the NIH was decreasing while that of PhD applicants was rapidly rising. In 1984 Gordon Gill of the University of California at San Diego published an essay ominously titled "The End of the Physician-Scientist?" He argued that those physicians who did continue to be engaged in research were increasingly drifting toward basic laboratory work, drawn by the irresistible appeal of the revolution in molecular biology. The clinician-scientist was becoming simply the "clinician-applier of basic science." The Nobel laureates Joseph Goldstein and Michael Brown, themselves prototypical physician-scientists, suggested that the movement of scientifically trained MDs toward basic research created a vacuum in clinical, patient-oriented research that was being filled by MDs who had neither the time to commit to research nor the required fundamental skills. Goldstein (1986) referred to such physicians, who typically lacked investigative creativity and courage, as having the "Paralyzed Academic Investigator's Disease Syndrome" or "PAIDS."

In response to the call for action, particularly emphasizing the need to revitalize clinically oriented research, several initiatives were undertaken beginning in the 1990s. In 1994 the Institute of Medicine published the outcome of its study on overcoming barriers to career paths for clinical research. In 1996 NIH director Harold Varmus commissioned an NIH task force, chaired by David G. Nathan, to propose recommendations to address the perceived shortfall of clinical investigators. The Nathan Committee found that the climate for clinical research performed by physician-scientists was in jeopardy of further deteriorating. Among its recommendations the committee supported the creation of new career development grants for patient-oriented research and loan repayment programs to assist clinical investigators in paying off their increasingly daunting educational debt. The Association of American Medical Colleges subsequently published reports of two task forces on clinical research, focusing again primarily on clinical (as opposed to basic laboratory) research performed by physician-scientists. Their recommendations included incorporating the underpinnings of clinical research in undergraduate and graduate medical education curricula and accelerating training in clinical research through comprehensive restructuring.

As the twentieth century drew to a close, new career development awards for physician-scientists from the NIH, as well as foundations such as the Burroughs Wellcome Fund, the Doris Duke Charitable Foundation, the Howard Hughes Medical Institute, and the Robert Wood Johnson Foundation, were targeted at revitalizing the physician-scientist workforce. (Outside the United States, organizations such as the Medical Research Council of the United Kingdom, INSERM in France, and the National Health and Medical Research Council of Australia developed similar programs.) These initiatives fortuitously coincided with a doubling of the NIH budget from about $14 billion in 1995 to $28 billion in 2003, raising the tide of confidence for young physicians contemplating research careers. Nevertheless, while there was an almost 50 percent increase among first-time PhD applicants for independent grants during the NIH budget-doubling period, the number of applicants with only MD degrees remained disappointingly flat. Indeed it has been essentially unchanged for over thirty years.

Today new challenges are fueling uncertainties about the future viability of the physician-scientist workforce. Beginning in 2003 the "un-doubling" of the NIH budget reinforced the perceived unpredictability of federal support for biomedical research, discouraging even more physicians from entering or staying in research careers when they have other, more secure career options available. Now, in 2009, the abrupt, dramatic, but very short-term and time-limited infusion of substantial amounts of new money into the NIH in response to the current economic crisis is unlikely to stimulate more physicians to enter research careers unless the increased support becomes meaningfully sustained. In addition, dramatic generational changes are occurring in the priorities of recent graduates of medical schools, including a desire for a more controllable lifestyle and greater balance between work and private demands. These generational differences in priorities may have profound implications for the future of academic medical research. Differences and tensions have begun to emerge between the current generation of mentors and their trainees. Finally, the impact of the recent disappearance of the gender gap among medical school graduates should be assessed in light of observations that, at least in the current academic environment, women find physician-scientist careers less attractive than do their male colleagues.

The Physician-Scientist Career Path

Currently the prototypical career path of a physician-scientist is long and arduous. In the United States, after four years of undergraduate college education and four years of medical school (or at least six years if both MD and PhD degrees are sought), the future physician-scientist is required to undertake several years of demanding, essentially full-time clinical training in a chosen field of practice. For example, for an internist who will specialize in cardiology, board eligibility requires three years of hospital residency in general internal medicine, followed by one to three additional years of clinical subspecialty training in cardiology. Following this prolonged full-time clinical training interlude, research training begins under the supervision of a designated faculty mentor. The typical duration of this period of intensive research experience is about two to four years, and it is often funded by either an institutional or individual research training grant. (When this support comes from the NIH, it is referred to as a "T"-type award.) There then follows a period of up to five years of progressively independent research, during which the young physician-scientist is gradually weaned from supervision by his or her mentor. Although a limited amount of time for clinical practice is encouraged during this stage, the majority of professional effort is typically devoted to research. While an initial medical school faculty appointment (at the instructor or assistant professor level) is usually made at this point, the young investigator is expected to compete successfully for extramural salary and research support to cover the research time. (When obtained from the NIH, these career development grants are in the form of "K" series awards.) Finally, the survivors of this process are able to obtain independent grant support (including the "R" series awards from the NIH, for example an RO1, often supplemented by other grants), enabling them to establish their own research operations, not infrequently at a different institution. The median age of investigators obtaining their first independent NIH RO1 grants has been progressively increasing, and is currently over forty-two. There is considerable controversy today about the need for such prolonged research training, creating opposing arguments by even the authors of this book.

This and other chapters in the book repeatedly refer to various types of research grant support from the NIH as the model metric for career success. While NIH funding has been widely regarded for the past half century in the United States as the "gold standard" for rigorously peer-reviewed, investigator-initiated medical research, it should be emphasized at this point in the introduction that many of the best training opportunities and greatest advances have been (and will undoubtedly continue to be) supported by other sources, including non-NIH government agencies, foundations, industry, and philanthropy. Indeed the career path of most productive physician-scientists is supported at different stages by a patchwork of grants from complementary and often opportunistic combinations of extramural sources.

Systems Biology

In addition to the sociological factors described so far, the apparently growing alienation of physicians from serious research careers largely parallels and reflects a widening schism between basic science and clinical medicine. In turn, the dramatic advances in molecular and cell biology in the second half of the twentieth century accelerated the reductionist approach to basic biomedical research. Indeed the emergence of ontological reductionism in biomedical research, already well developed in the physical sciences, does not practically require the involvement of physicians at all.

To counterbalance this trend, the field of "systems biology" has arisen in recent years. Systems biology in medical research is directed at studying the complex interactions that occur in whole biological systems. It applies rigorous data integration and mathematical models to a holistic analysis of biological networks. As Denis Noble (2006) described it, systems biology "is about putting together rather than taking apart, integration rather than reduction." Some have used the analogy of studying an automobile. It is not possible to understand how a car works, much less be able to service it when it malfunctions, by focusing only on its taillights or seatbelts or transmission in isolation. In this way it can be anticipated that systems biology will reanimate the critical link between basic biomedical research and the clinical study of disease.

Translational Research

Today, reinforcing this link has become vital. The last decades of the twentieth century witnessed not only an explosive growth in our knowledge of molecular biology but also, simultaneously, the mushrooming complexity of clinical practice. As a result, the divide that separates fundamental biomedical research from advances in improving the health of human individuals and populations has become a rapidly widening abyss. A veritable language barrier has developed between basic scientists and practitioners of clinical medicine. Attempts to bridge this chasm have created a new term, "translational research." Interestingly, the term first appeared in the medical literature (PubMed) as recently as 1993, was mentioned in only a handful of articles annually until about 2000, and then rapidly proliferated, with references to it currently in several thousand papers each year. Entire new journals are now dedicated to the topic; many universities are developing advanced degree programs in translational research; and major new governmental funding streams (e.g., the Clinical and Translational Science Awards of the National Institutes of Health) have been implemented.

Yet in effect, translational research has been around for more than a century. In the early 1900s it primarily took the form of "bedside-to-bench" investigation. This was because medical research at that time was dominated by actively practicing physicians. The most inquisitive of these "naturalists" extended their keen observations of patients to experimentation that might reveal fundamental mechanisms of disease. Indeed, as Goldstein (1986) has pointed out, the hallmark of an outstanding physician-as-scientist is having the "technical courage" to master whatever experimental methods are needed to be able to answer basic questions raised in the course of caring for patients. (Today, faced with a daunting repertoire of highly technical laboratory methods that no single investigator can ever hope to command, it is often sufficient for "bedside-to-bench" physician-scientists to seek and identify scientific collaborators with the appropriate technical expertise to help them answer questions inspired by their clinical observations. This problem-based investigator mentality is more intellectually rewarding than the reverse, that is, the technique-based investigator approach of possessing mastery of a single laboratory skill and then searching for clinical questions to which it can be applied.)

In the second half of the twentieth century, the great expansion in the number of PhD basic biomedical scientists created a reversal of the predominant direction of translational research to one of "bench-to-bedside." Here medical discoveries originated in the laboratory, and it was left up to mostly physician-scientists to attempt to apply them to patient care or to commercialize them ("bring them to market"). Truly effective translational research in the future will require a rebalancing of its direction to one of a dynamic, continuously streaming transit back and forth between bench and bedside.

Finally, we now understand that translational research cannot be limited to a bidirectional flow between the laboratory and the individual patient. Indeed the pathway of clinical research must extend to the health of the population: bench-to-bedside-to-populations and the reverse. (That this stage of the clinical research continuum is not acknowledged by some to be strictly part of the translational research enterprise reflects a lack of unanimity about the definition of "translational medicine.")

Barriers in Translational Research

Major barriers in the translational research continuum occur not only in the transfer of research knowledge between the laboratory and the individual patient but also in its translation from individual patient care into everyday decision making in clinical practice and its penetration to improving the health of the population. These "translational blocks," identified by the Clinical Research Roundtable that was convened by the Institute of Medicine in 2000, are depicted in figure 0.1.

The skills needed today to conduct productive basic laboratory research include mastery of molecular biology, genetics, animal models of disease, and often specialized expertise in areas such as biomedical engineering and the physical sciences. This workforce has been increasingly populated by PhD scientists and physician-scientists who have become largely detached from clinical practice. The skills needed to do patient-oriented clinical research include clinical trials design, biostatistics and clinical informatics, phenotyping and biobanking methods, and at least a strong understanding of laboratory science. This workforce is composed primarily of

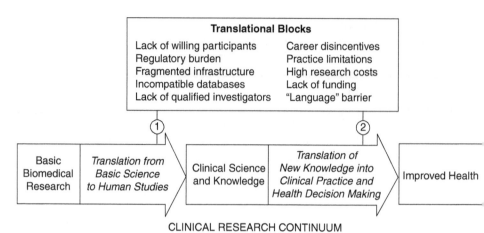

Figure 0.1. The causes and sites of "translational blocks" in the continuum of clinical research (modified from Sung, Crowley, Genel et al. 2003).

clinically active physician-scientists and other nonphysician health professionals. And the skills required to conduct population-based evaluative research include diverse disciplines such as clinical epidemiology, public health, behavioral and social sciences, computational biology, health policy, and economics. Individual investigators in this field can be either physician-scientists, PhD scholars specializing in these areas, or even non–health care professionals.

While the central premise of this book is that physicians must continue to play a vital, irreplaceable, and leading role in the medical research enterprise of the future, the involvement of nonphysician scientists, particularly those with PhD degrees, is becoming ever more critical. Combined MD-PhD training programs are thriving, and the number of pure PhD faculty members in clinical departments has been growing at a faster rate than that of any other faculty group in American medical schools. Innovative graduate programs have begun to develop curricula to introduce PhD students formally to the world of clinical medicine. The power of the complementary perspectives that clinical investigators and basic scientists can bring to medical research should more than offset traditional cultural barriers between them. In fact, when the Nobel laureate George Hoyt Whipple became the founding dean of the University of Rochester Medical School, he designed a curriculum in the 1920s that involved co-training of medical students and predoctoral students. In his book *The Crisis in Clinical Research*, Edward Ahrens (1992) wondered "whether young MDs and PhDs are not ideally equipped to train each other."

The Evolution of Physicians as Members
of Research Teams

It is axiomatic, then, that in the future, the continuing extraordinary growth of both basic biomedical science and clinical knowledge will make it impossible for any one individual to single-handedly navigate the entire bidirectional path between bench, bedside, and populations. The solitary, versatile physician-scientist of an earlier time is now largely obsolete. The medical science of tomorrow will require, much more than in the past, the dynamic assembly of multidisciplinary teams of researchers. As physicians (and other scientists) become ever more narrowly specialized in their expertise, breadth in medical research will be attained only through hand-in-glove collaborations. This new organizational paradigm for medical research raises important questions, however. Without a strong leader, the collaborating team is likely to lose its bearings and even disintegrate. So who is best qualified to lead such complex teams of investigators to ensure that they remain well coordinated, integrated, and on track? How will individual investigators who make major contributions to a team receive recognition as leaders (or "principal investigators")? Where will the physician-scientist of tomorrow best fit into the teams that traverse the path of medical research?

Figure 0.2 envisions an idealized bidirectional highway of medical research. It spans the extensive continuum from basic to clinical to population-based investigation. In fact at the "basic end" it even extends, without limit, into the physical sciences and engineering, while at the "populations end" it stretches and divides into more distant social sciences. The highway has innumerable exit and entrance ramps that connect with networks of side roads. These represent the rich digressions (perhaps "scenic detours" and sometimes even "dead ends") that are so essential to inspire creativity, innovation, and risk taking in medical research; but they must all be able to return ultimately to the main highway in order to maintain the unwavering focus of the medical research enterprise on human health. Vehicles on the side roads must never lose sight of the main highway. The vehicles (research teams) that traverse the highway in either direction vary in the number and composition of passengers (investigators); they pick up and discharge passengers and even change drivers (principal investigators) at different way stations. At some stages of the journey, particularly at the basic end, vehicles may contain few (or even no) MD investigators, while at others, particularly around the clinical area, they will contain mostly (or all) MD investigators. It will be virtually impossible for any one individual to know the directions (expertise), to be the driver, or even to be one of

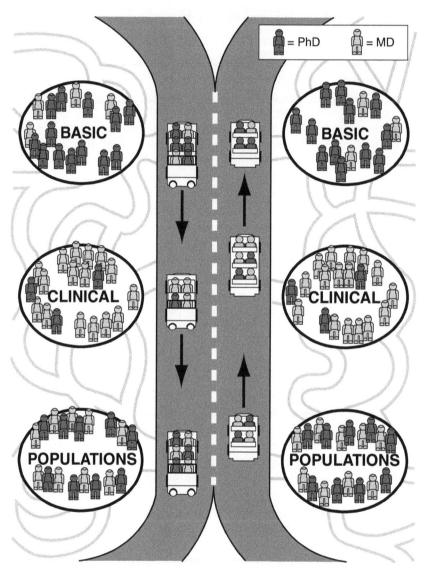

Figure 0.2. The schematic two-way highway of medical research, spanning the continuum from basic to clinical to population-based research and beyond. Teams of investigators, including physician-scientists, traverse the highway in both directions, driven in cars containing varying numbers and types of researchers, depending on expertise required at different stages. The model is described in greater detail in the text.

the passengers for the entire length of the research highway. The dynamic composition of an effective medical research team of the future will always need an expert driver to ensure that it does not get lost, but it will also provide the opportunity for scientists of different backgrounds, certainly including physician-scientists, to take the wheel at different stages of the journey. And each passenger plays a vital role, whether it be reading the map, fixing a flat tire, pointing out road hazards, relieving a sleepy driver, or filling the car with gas.

It has been suggested that the "big science" of tomorrow will require the organization of sometimes enormous research consortia. Note that the vehicles shown in figure 0.2, however, are cars, not buses. This is because, as articulated by the pioneering cancer biologist Robert Weinberg (2006), much of the most innovative and influential medical research will undoubtedly continue to emerge from "relatively small, highly mobile, creative research groups" that operate opportunistically.

Consider the following fictitious (but not unrealistic) sequence of medical discoveries. An astute practicing physician makes a striking observation in one of his patients who is dying of a rare cancer which has not responded to any kind of known treatment. After the patient starts to take a new drug to treat his unrelated coronary heart disease, the tumor begins to shrink. The physician doesn't know if this is a fortuitous coincidence or a totally unexpected effect of the heart drug. So the drug is taken to the laboratory to test its effects on a piece of tumor tissue that had been saved from the patient's original biopsy ("bedside-to-bench" research). The drug indeed stops the growth of the cancer cells in a test tube. It is discovered in further experiments that the heart drug works by blocking a specific molecular reaction in the tumor. This reaction is then found to be linked to a group of enzymes in the tumor cells called TAM receptor tyrosine kinases; these enzymes were previously known to go haywire in this particular cancer. Experiments are then performed that isolate a very powerful and specific small molecule, TAM tyrosine kinase inhibitor. The new drug is tested in genetically altered mice that have the same kind of cancer, and it is found to be effective. Large-scale drug development of this inhibitor is started, leading to clinical trials in patients with the cancer ("bench-to-bedside" research). The drug works well, but only in about 10 percent of the patients, and it causes some significant side effects. It is approved for use by the Food and Drug Administration, but it is extremely expensive. Research must now be done to demonstrate its cost effectiveness, identify which subgroups of patients with this cancer best respond to the drug, and determine how to get it to medically underserved populations.

It is practically impossible for any one physician-scientist to have the expertise and resources to participate in all phases of this research. But he can become involved in some parts. In fact he could even drive certain stages of the journey. For example, he might have made the original clinical observation that started the trail of discovery in the first place. And then, when it comes back to him from the laboratory, the same physician could become the principal investigator of a Phase III randomized clinical trial to test the effectiveness of the new drug in patients with this form of cancer. Another scientist, working elsewhere, who is a highly specialized expert in TAM tyrosine kinases and TAM receptor signaling pathways, might have led the team that developed the inhibitor drug. Other groups of investigators are likely to come to this scientist to test targeted inhibition of TAM receptor tyrosine kinases for other diseases, such as autoimmune disorders, vascular diseases, and other types of cancer. And so physician-scientists and nonphysician-scientists will continue to make enormous personal contributions to research teams as they that travel up and down different stages of tomorrow's highway of medical discovery. In order to continue this tradition of discovery, however, it will be essential to ensure an adequate supply of physicians who want to work as scientists.

Roadmap

In the subsequent chapters prominent scholars describe and analyze the breadth of the challenges facing this particular research population of investigators. They consider the forces that have created and fueled the current crisis and propose workable solutions that can help reinvigorate the physician-scientist workforce. The first chapter describes the history of the physician as scientist and explores the major contributions physicians have made to scientific knowledge and patient care. In the second chapter Timothy Ley presents a statistical investigation of the physician-scientist workforce, describing where it has been and where it is going. In chapter 3 David Korn and Stephen Heinig give us an in-depth understanding of the ecology of the physician-scientist in academic medicine. "Translational research" is the centerpiece of the physician-scientist's role in the medical research enterprise as described in chapter 4 by Barry Coller.

In chapter 5 Reshma Jagsi and Nancy Tarbell outline the particular problems women encounter as they move through careers in academic medicine and make concrete suggestions that would positively impact the number of women who embark on a career as physician-scientists. Chapters 6 and 7 then consider two vexing problems and enormous opportunities that new generational cohorts bring to medical research: Ann Brown suggests interesting ways to approach the striking differences between baby boomers, generation Xers, and millennials, while Stephen Emerson and his colleagues at Haverford College describe an example of a program designed to interest undergraduates in physician-scientist careers.

The next chapters move into more programmatic and institutional analyses for dealing with the challenges to the physician-scientist workforce. Philip Pizzo describes the relationship between academic medical centers and the cultivation of the physician as scientist. In chapter 9 Roy Silverstein and Paul DiCorleto then explore how to optimize the relationships between physicians and PhD scientists involved in medical research.

Strong mentorship will be more critical than ever to the creation of the next generation of physician-scientists. In chapters 10 and 11 Kenneth Kaushansky, Alan Schwartz, and Margaret Hostetter deal with the issue of how to mentor new generations of physicians in ways that will help them navigate the long and difficult road that leads to a successful research career. In Chapter 12 Mark Donowitz and his colleagues focus on the financial ramifications of the physician-scientist career and make specific recommendations directed to academic medical centers and the National Institutes of Health.

David Korn and Stephen Heinig return in chapter 13 to describe how the Association of American Medical Colleges is dealing with the challenges of restoring and invigorating the physician-scientist workforce. In chapter 14 I continue this discussion by presenting the detailed suggestions made by the Association of Professors of Medicine, which has launched a major initiative designed to ensure that physicians as scientists will continue to advance knowledge and patient care in the decades to come.

To conclude, one of the country's most prominent physician-scientists, David Nathan, has written an eloquent essay on the challenges he has confronted and opportunities he has found in the course of his own influential career. We hope that it will inspire young physicians to embark on this rewarding career while inspiring more established researchers to celebrate the work of future generations of physician-scientists whose careers they will have been in the enviable position to shape.

Although this book is devoted to transforming the environment that produces and nourishes physicians as scientists, it is clear that the exact form in which physicians will be engaged in research in the future cannot be expected to remain unchanged. Many today who lament the apparent decline in interest of physicians in medical research cling to the Oslerian ideal of the individual clinical investigator who can by himself or herself shuttle effortlessly back and forth between bedside and bench, managing both a busy clinical practice and a productive research laboratory. The greatly admired prototypical "triple threat" academic physician of the twentieth century, who could independently juggle major clinical, research, and teaching responsibilities during the course of the day, is not likely to be the most effective model of the physician-scientist in tomorrow's world of increasingly complex clinical practice and rapidly advancing biomedical knowledge. We do not and cannot know what form the role of the physician-scientist will take in the future. But it is reassuring that the history of the physician as scientist reflects the enduring but continually changing models of involvement of physicians in the medical research enterprise.

1

History of the Physician as Scientist

Andrew I. Schafer, MD

While physicians have played a pivotal, often leading role in medical investigation throughout history, the manner of their involvement in the research enterprise has evolved over time. As the ability or even necessity of physicians also to function as scientists is increasingly questioned in today's era of extraordinarily rapid advances in the biomedical sciences, it is instructive to begin the discussion with a historical perspective. In this chapter I first illustrate why and how physicians have pioneered many of the great breakthroughs in medical science, and then provide an overview of their central but ever-changing role in the medical research enterprise throughout history.

Physician Pioneers in Medical Research

The Nobel Prize in Medicine

Since the first Nobel Prizes were awarded in 1901, 103 of the 189 laureates in physiology or medicine have been physicians (Shalev 2005). Ten other physicians have won the Nobel Prize in chemistry or physics. Several of them are referred to in more detail later in the chapter, including Pavlov, Koch, Ehrlich, and Fleming. Others include Golgi, leader in exploring the structure of the nervous system; Banting, co-discoverer of insulin; Landsteiner, discoverer of human blood groups; Warburg, pioneer of respiratory enzymes; both Coris, who elucidated glycogenolysis; Krebs, discoverer of the citric acid cycle; Kornberg and Ochoa, who demonstrated how DNA and RNA are synthesized; Rous, discoverer of tumor-inducing viruses; Brown and Goldstein, who demonstrated cholesterol metabolism; and Bishop and Varmus, pioneers in oncogene research (Shalev 2005). Notably, while 80 percent of the laureates in medicine during the first four decades of the Nobel Prize were physicians, sixteen of the twenty from 2001 to 2008 were PhDs, reflecting trends that are discussed later in this chapter.

Practicing Physicians Breaking Ground

The impact of physicians in advancing medical science is not limited to those who have devoted their careers to research. History is replete with examples of practicing clinicians, untrained in research, who have made astute observations of patients that led to important discoveries. In many cases these practitioners themselves pursued their clinical observations into the laboratory; in others their extraordinary clinical insights stimulated the work of established scientists to create the medical breakthrough.

Edward Jenner was a country doctor in Berkeley, a village in Gloucestershire, England. He had studied medicine in London under John Hunter, the great English surgeon and naturalist, who became a lifelong friend. He felt uncomfortable in the city, however, and returned to his idyllic town of birth. There he might have lived out his life in blissful obscurity had it not been for his insatiable curiosity, no doubt inspired in part by regular communication with Hunter. Smallpox had been a scourge of mankind since antiquity, dating back to at least ancient Egypt. Jenner was well aware of the practice of variolation or "engrafting," popularized in the early eighteenth century by Lady Mary Wortley Montagu, the wife of the British ambassador to Constantinople, a great beauty who had herself become disfigured by smallpox.

Variolation was intended to prevent full-blown cases by exposing individuals to the disease by scratching the skin with a pin that had been introduced into a sore in a patient with active smallpox. Variolation had been administered to Jenner himself when he was a young boy. The treatment, however, was impractical to implement on a large scale and had a high mortality rate. Now, while pursuing his general practice career, Jenner began to observe and record the cases of milkmaids in Gloucestershire, who were noted for their clear complexions. They had apparently acquired lifetime protection from smallpox by contracting cases of the much milder disease cowpox in the course of their work. By 1796 Jenner was ready to test his observations experimentally, encouraged in letters from his friend Hunter. On May 14 he transferred pus from a sore on the hand of Sarah Nelmes, a milkmaid suffering from cowpox, into incisions he made in an eight-year-old boy named James Phipps. James developed some relatively mild symptoms but promptly recovered. Six weeks later Jenner injected James with pus taken from a patient with active smallpox, and the boy remained well; indeed Jenner repeated the exposure several months later, again with no ill effects. Despite his subsequent ability to reproduce successful vaccination in a number of subjects, Jenner's findings were originally met with great skepticism from the medical establishment and condemnation by the clergy. While understanding the mechanism of vaccination would have to await the germ theory of disease in the next century, Edward Jenner's keen observations and curiosity would pave the way for the first eradication of an infectious disease, as certified by the World Health Organization in 1980.

Physicians also greatly advanced the understanding and treatment of cholera. Repeated epidemics of the deadly Asian form of the disease swept England and Europe in the early nineteenth century, decimating populations. Cholera typically struck healthy individuals, often leading to their terrifying death within hours. Without any insight into its cause or treatment, physicians were powerless. The accepted forms of supportive management almost certainly hastened rather than ameliorated the course of the illness. They included bleeding (whenever it was possible to do so from the collapsed veins of moribund patients), castor oil for diarrhea, and emetics to induce vomiting. The mode of transmission of cholera was likewise entirely unknown, although there was no dearth of theories: malodorous gases, "effluvia" emitted from the bodies of victims, even underlying geological phenomena, or, as Robert Adler described it, "a combination of out-of-whack bodily humors and exposure to miasmas" (Adler 2004).

Then, within a period of less than twenty-five years, in the course of two successive outbreaks of cholera in England, three physicians with virtually no training in research separately broke open our understanding of the mode of transmission and treatment of cholera. William Brooke O'Shaughnessy, a resourceful young Irishman, went to London immediately after graduating from Edinburgh's medical school, but was barred from practicing medicine by the rigidly closed franchise of London physicians. To make a living, he opened a forensic toxicology laboratory to perform chemical analyses of bodily fluids and tissues for hospitals, physicians, and courts. When the second pandemic of Asian cholera struck in the port of Sunderland, in northeast England, in the fall of 1831, O'Shaughnessy traveled to the epicenter and carried out meticulous and detailed chemical analyses of the blood, emesis, and diarrhea of cholera victims.

He demonstrated how the profuse diarrhea of the disease causes profound dehydration, electrolyte imbalance, acidosis, and uremia. In his article in the *Lancet* he concluded that effective treatment should require "first, to restore the blood to its natural water content; secondly, to restore its deficient saline matters." O'Shaughnessy went so far as to perform experiments of intravenous resuscitation in dogs. It remained for Thomas Latta, however, an established general practitioner in Leith, to apply O'Shaughnessy's findings to human subjects with cholera. He was unsuccessful in replenishing fluids and electrolytes orally or by enema. Therefore, as he later wrote in his *Lancet* paper in 1832, he "at length resolved to throw the fluid immediately into the circulation" via an intravenous tube inserted into the basilic vein. Latta achieved some dramatic successes but also many failures, probably because the saline infusions were not maintained long enough and were given only in the terminal stages of the illness. When the cholera pandemic subsided in 1832, the work of these two insightful doctors was largely forgotten until it was reintroduced by Little, Barnes, and Schwarz in the 1880s. But the perseverance and resourcefulness of these physicians actually pioneered the field of fluid resuscitation and intravenous therapy (Baskett 2002).

When cholera again invaded England in 1848, it fell on a busy practitioner named John Snow to make an extraordinary breakthrough. Snow, who practiced surgery, had become a leading anesthetist in the Soho district of London. He was described as a "keen and careful observer, an astute diagnostician, and a caring and careful physician." As such, he had challenged the prevailing theory of transmission of cholera by the inhalation of putrid gases referred to as "miasma," arguing that the disease affected the intestines, not the lungs. Indeed Snow hypothesized that cholera was spread by fecal contamination of drinking water. When the English cholera epidemic invaded his Soho neighborhood, he made the observation that nearly all of its victims there had used water from a common pump on Broad Street. Furthermore, Snow noted that workers in a brewery on the same street, which had its own water well, were spared, as were the convicts in a neighborhood prison, who likewise did not use the Broad Street pump. Despite local opposition, Snow persuaded desperate city officials to disconnect the pump. This intervention immediately resulted in a precipitous decline in cases. While Snow's conclusions antedated the germ theory of disease by a generation, the observations of this practicing surgeon, and his follow-up studies, essentially opened the field of epidemiology.

The same type of keen clinical insight transformed the experience of women in childbirth. Shortly after his graduation from medical school in

1844, the Hungarian obstetrician Ignac Semmelweis was appointed assistant to Professor Johann Klein, the politically well connected "old guard" chief of the large lying-in unit of Vienna's Allgemeine Krankenhaus. This obstetrical service was ravaged at that time by an epidemic of puerperal fever, also known as childbed fever, which was taking the lives of one of every six mothers delivered in the First Division of the hospital. While its cause was unknown, autopsies of women who had succumbed to the disease invariably revealed pools and pockets of fetid fluid and pus in their abdominal cavities, associated with extensive swelling and inflammation of the female organs. The young Semmelweis became virtually obsessed with the problem. He put together several key observations. First, the number of deliveries was about equally divided between the First and Second Divisions of the hospital's obstetrical services. The only difference was that deliveries in the First Division were carried out by teaching physicians and medical students, while those in the Second Division were done by midwives. The mortality rate due to puerperal fever was about 10 percent in the First Division but less than 4 percent in the Second Division. Second, there was no epidemic outside the hospital walls, and in fact death from puerperal fever was exceedingly rare in women who delivered at home or even in alleyways and streets. Third, in contrast to many other epidemics, the mortality rate from puerperal fever was unrelated to weather.

Semmelweis seized on the critical difference between the divisions. The medical students and attending physicians on the First Division—but not the midwives on the Second Division—would routinely walk straight from their autopsy exercises to examine the women in labor on the wards, without changing their clothing and after washing their hands only perfunctorily if at all. Yet their autopsies typically involved dissecting the bodies of women who had just died from puerperal fever. In the words of Semmelweis himself, "puerperal fever was nothing more nor less than cadaveric blood poisoning." As Sherwin Nuland commented in his book *The Doctors' Plague* (Nuland 2003), "among the most critical of the qualities characterizing the successful researcher is the ability to separate wheat from chaff," to sort out the critical observations from the wealth of data on which a discovery must be based. And here, as Nuland notes, "Semmelweis was unerring in his accuracy." Tragically, the simple solution of demanding that physicians and students wash their hands before examining patients was considered a subversive idea in the reactionary medical community of the Vienna of that time. Semmelweis was ridiculed, ostracized, and ultimately banished to Budapest, where he died in an insane asylum. But this young practitioner's keen observations and perseverance were subsequently vindicated by the work of Pasteur, Koch, Lister, and others in the development of the germ theory and the practice of antisepsis.

Some of the key developments in modern cardiac pathophysiology originated with the keen observations of general practitioners. In the nineteenth century, many people were rendered cardiac invalids by their doctors who had discovered them to have irregular heartbeats. James Mackenzie, an Edinburgh medical school graduate, was engaged in a busy group general practice in the industrial city of Burnley in northern England. Despite an enormous clinical workload, he was a meticulous observer and careful note taker. To understand the extra systolic heartbeats he discovered in his patients, he developed the polygraph, which enabled him to diagnose various forms of heart block. Following patients over long periods, he was able to distinguish the benign course of many types of cardiac arrhythmias and murmurs. Mackenzie thus laid the foundation for modern cardiac electrophysiology. Paul Dudley White later referred to him as the "father" of modern cardiology.

Lawrence Craven, a suburban general practitioner in Glendale, California, is now belatedly recognized for having made the original, albeit uncontrolled, observations that led to the discovery of the antithrombotic effects of aspirin. Craven, who had performed hundreds of tonsillectomies in his practice, noted in the 1940s that an "alarming number of hemorrhages" began to occur "in disturbing frequency" (Milner 2007). He linked these bleeding complications to the chewing of aspirin gum to relieve pain, and made the conceptual leap in a letter to the *Annals of Western Medicine and Surgery* in 1950 that aspirin could therefore prevent coronary thrombosis. He began to prescribe daily aspirin to his male patients who were between the ages of forty-five and sixty-five, were overweight, and led sedentary lifestyles, and reported in a 1953 paper in the *Mississippi Valley Medical Journal* that none of them had suffered a myocardial infarction over several years of follow-up. Craven never trained as a scientist, and he humbly acknowledged his limitations. Yet this single clinician's remarkable insights set the stage for the pharmacologic revolution in preventive cardiology.

For each such story of transformative discoveries by practicing physicians there are countless others in which clinical observations have contributed to the foundations of modern medical science. In a 1931 lecture to the Cambridge University Medical Society titled "The Physician as Scientist and Naturalist," the physician John Ryle noted that the physician is first and foremost a student of nature, observing, recording, classifying, and analyzing. Ryle remarked that "the naturalistic temperament and the physicianly temperament are, as we should imagine, close relations, if not identical twins" (Ryle 1999).

Physicians as Experimental Subjects

Throughout history, physician-investigators have been matchlessly positioned to experiment on themselves. Despite the altruistic motives that have often driven self-experimentation, ethical reservations about the practice have been repeatedly raised. Indeed there are many stories of misguided, even reckless and nutty experiments by physicians and medical students, fictionalized in books such as Robert Louis Stevenson's *Strange Case of Dr. Jekyll and Mr. Hyde* and *The Invisible Man* by H. G. Wells. Nevertheless, as Lawrence Altman has pointed out in his book *Who Goes First?*, "in a long and continuing tradition, many doctors have chosen to be the first volunteer, believing that it is the most ethical way to accept responsibility for the unknown risks associated with the first steps in human experimentation" (Altman 1998).

There are numerous stories of success, often coming at a high price to the health and even the life of the physician-investigator. In 1767 John Hunter, Jenner's mentor, infected himself with gonorrhea and syphilis by self-injection from a prostitute with both diseases: many years later he died of a probable dissection of a syphilitic aortic aneurysm. In 1885 a Peruvian medical student named Daniel Carrión died from progressive anemia in the process of proving the cause of an infectious disease called bartonellosis after injecting himself, with the help of colleagues, with material from the skin lesion of a patient. In 1900 three physician members of Walter Reed's team in Cuba (but, contrary to legend, not Reed himself) proved that mosquitoes transmit the microbe that causes yellow fever by applying to their own skin mosquitoes that had previously fed on patients with the disease; at least one and possibly two of the team members died as a consequence. In 1929 Werner Forssman courageously conducted the first series of cardiac catheterizations on himself, using a ureteral (urinary) catheter that he inserted into a vein in his arm and then threaded up into the interior of his heart. In 1950 William Harrington, in collaboration with a fellow hematology colleague, James Hollingsworth, demonstrated that some factor in blood plasma (later proven to be an antibody) causes the self-destruction of blood platelets in a serious bleeding disorder called idiopathic thrombocytopenic purpura (ITP). He proved the hypothesis by having a pint of blood transfused into himself from a patient with ITP. This led to a precipitous decline in his own platelet count, nearly causing his death from internal bleeding. In 1985 Barry Marshall swallowed a solution of *Helicobacter pylori*, then had his own stomach endoscoped and biopsied to prove that this bacterium causes gastritis and ulcers. Even as recently as 2007, Craig Venter announced that he had fully sequenced the entire (6 billion–letter) human genome using his own DNA, and breaking the privacy taboo of revealing his own disease susceptibilities.

These and other examples of human self-experimentation have led to some revolutionary insights into certain areas of medicine, such as cardio-vascular physiology, infectious diseases, the development of anesthesia, peptic ulcer disease, and autoimmune disorders.

The Evolution of the Physician-Scientist

Antiquity and the Middle Ages

Transcendental and supernatural beliefs in the character of illness began to be replaced by natural explanation during Graeco-Roman antiquity and the great Asian civilizations. Hippocrates (ca. 460–377 BCE), the most cele-brated physician in history, is considered by many to be the first clinician-scientist. Central to Hippocratic thinking was the concept of health as equilibrium and illness as disorder. And these principles were rooted in his teaching that the practice of medicine must depend on careful, pains-taking observation of patients and the application of reason. Hippocrates and his students had to rely on the surface observation of human anat-omy, as dissection was forbidden. Observational medical science flour-ished in the Hellenistic world for a very brief period after Hippocrates. Two physicians, Herophilus (ca. 330–260 BCE) and his rival Erasistratus (ca. 330–255 BCE), founders of the great medical school in Alexandria, laid the foundations of human anatomy and physiology by exploring for the first time what lay inside the human body. But they did not have students who could carry on their brilliant studies.

Galen (129–ca. 216 CE) began his medical career as a physician to gladi-ators, which provided him with ample opportunities to make anatomi-cal and physiological observations in the course of treatment of traumatic injuries. While human dissection was forbidden, Galen vivisected ani-mals, including primates. He made brilliant physiological discoveries by experimenting with severing the spinal cords of living animals at different levels and tying off blood vessels to prove that blood flows outward from the heart. A prolific but bombastic, arrogant, and egotistical physician-investigator (who once wrote, "It is I, and I alone, who have revealed the true path of medicine"), Galen became the foremost medical celebrity of ancient Rome. Although he was an experimental genius, Galen could not resist expanding his incisive scientific observations into a grand scheme of human health, disease, and temperament shaped by the dogma of hu-mors. Ironically, Galenic doctrine was to paralyze medical progress for the next fifteen hundred years.

For medical science the Dark Ages after Galen extended into the Renaissance with precious few bright lights. One of them, uncovered in the West only in the twentieth century, was the great Islamic surgeon Ibn al-Nafis (ca. 1210–1288). While he denied performing dissections, which were prohibited by Islamic law, al-Nafis courageously challenged Galenic dogma and made remarkable anatomic discoveries. Most notably, he wrote that it was impossible for blood to flow directly from one side of the heart to the other, and thus ascertained the existence of a heart-lung circulation. But in general, the Middle Ages, mired in wars and plagues, lost touch with the science and rationalism of ancient Greece and Rome.

The Renaissance

Among the first to emerge from this barren millennium for medical science was an eccentric and grandiose Swiss rebel who named himself Paracelsus (meaning "greater than Celsus," the famous ancient Roman medical encyclopedist). Paracelsus (1493–1541) practiced medicine despite a highly dubious medical education. Throughout his life he wandered all over Europe, contemptuously and combatively alienating the local medical establishment wherever he went. Nevertheless, Paracelsus made the first notable assault on the foundations of Galenic medicine. He argued that each disease must have a unique cause and cure. He also disdained the traditional use of complex potions that could not be tested for efficacy and predicted that chemistry would create pure drugs to target specific diseases. In many ways he was the founder of medical chemistry.

Two years after the death of Paracelsus, Andreas Vesalius (1514–1564) of Padua published his monumental anatomical atlas, *De Humani Corporis Fabrica*. Vesalius studied medicine at the University of Paris, but political turmoil forced him to leave France; he was later awarded his medical degree by the University of Padua. Unlike generations of medical professors before him, who considered human dissection vulgar and delegated the task to barber-surgeon assistants while they lectured on Galen's unchallenged writings, Vesalius performed innumerable human dissections himself. He also did his own laboratory experiments. Galen, as Vesalius wrote, "never dissected the body of a man who had recently died." Thereafter medicine would be rooted in an accurate knowledge of human anatomy based on systematic firsthand dissection. Robert Adler has noted that "along with a few other Renaissance giants such as Copernicus and Galileo, Vesalius created the progressive, science-driven world in which we live" (Adler 2004). After publication of the *Fabrica*, Vesalius became a full-time clinician and was appointed imperial physician to Emperor Charles V.

If Vesalius laid the foundation of medicine as an "observational science," William Harvey (1578–1657) laid its foundation as a "functional science." Likewise educated in medicine at the University of Padua, Harvey returned to his native England, received an appointment at St. Batholomew's Hospital, and launched a successful career in the practice of medicine among the elite of London. He later became royal physician to King James I and King Charles I. While maintaining his busy practice, Harvey devoted considerable time to extensive anatomical studies of humans and animals. In demonstrating the circulation of the blood, Harvey built on the anatomy of Vesalius. He showed, however, that observation (which he did in fact greatly value) was not sufficient: it must be followed by physiological experimentation. Furthermore, Harvey introduced quantitative analysis as an integral part of medical experimentation. The revolutionary work of this classical physician-scientist, epitomized in his masterpiece, *De Motu Cordis*, not only demonstrated the circulation as a "circle in a state of ceaseless motion" pumped by the heart but also inspired those who followed him to use experimentation and quantitative reasoning in medical research.

Because he did not have a microscope, one important gap remained in Harvey's model of the circulation: he could not see the microvascular connection between arteries and veins. The microscope was developed by nonphysician scientists. It was originally constructed by Dutch spectacle makers around 1600, then most productively applied by others, including the Dutchman Anton van Leeuwenhoek (1632–1723), a cloth merchant and wine taster by trade, and Robert Hooke (1634–1703), an English physicist. It was left to the Italian physician Marcello Malpighi (1628–1694), using this instrument, to close the loop three years after Newton's death by directly visualizing capillaries perfused by red blood cells.

Rise of the Research Tradition

By the early nineteenth century, most European countries had developed medical schools staffed by physician faculty who assumed substantial academic responsibilities. England lagged behind, with much of the medical education there carried out in private anatomy schools. English students who sought a more academic medical education went north to the Scottish schools in Edinburgh and Glasgow. Later in the nineteenth century, English medical schools arose connected to hospitals, patterned after the hospital-based French schools that emphasized the importance of careful physical diagnosis and autopsies. The French model of medical education was epitomized by René Laënnec (1781–1826), who invented the stethoscope and used this instrument to diagnose diseases of the heart and lungs that would subsequently be correlated with autopsy findings.

The requirement of incorporating laboratory experience in the training of all physicians was first established by the middle of the nineteenth century in the German schools. In contrast to the schools of France and England that were attached to hospitals, the German medical school was firmly established in the university. In this way German university-based medical schools were the first to cultivate the ethos of research in medicine. In the German medical school the laboratory, not the hospital, became the center of discovery; the microscope, not the stethoscope, became the main instrument for learning. By the second half of the nineteenth century, great medical research institutes flourished in conjunction with universities in Germany. These growing research centers were generously supported, and their physician professors were afforded ample time away from clinical work to pursue research and teaching.

Many of the greatest physician-scientists of the late nineteenth and early twentieth centuries were incubated in this intellectually vibrant environment for medical research. Where there is such a purposeful confluence of protected time to work within a robust culture of research, academic freedom, ample and stable funding, and an intellectual critical mass, research and teaching become inextricably connected.

No better example of the power of strong mentoring can be found than the remarkable genealogy of physician-investigators that can be traced back to Johannes Peter Müller (1801–1858). Müller excelled in his medical studies at the University of Bonn, quickly rose there through the faculty ranks to full professorship, and by the age of thirty-two had received the coveted professorship of anatomy, physiology, and pathology at the University of Berlin. Müller's output of original work in neurophysiology, microscopic and embryonic anatomy, and pathological histology was prodigious. Those who flocked to his laboratory to study under him included Carl Ludwig (1816–1895), who subsequently made groundbreaking contributions to the physiology of blood pressure, urinary excretion, and anesthesia, and later founded the renowned Ludwig Institute of Physiology in Leipzig; Hermann Helmholtz (1821–1894), pioneer of physiological optics, electricity, and magnetism; Emil du Bois-Reymond (1818–1896), the founder of modern electrophysiology; Theodor Schwann (1810–1882), who founded modern histology by defining the cell as the basic unit of animal tissue; Friedrich Gustav Jakob Henle (1809–1885), pioneer of cytology, discoverer of the loop of Henle in the kidney, and one of the original thinkers of the germ theory of disease; Ernst Haeckel (1834–1919), who coined the term "ontogeny recapitulates phylogeny"; Ernst Wilhelm von Brücke (1819–1892), one of the originators of cellular physiology; and Rudolf Virchow (1821–1902), the father of modern cellular pathology. All of these students were physicians by training. Each of them in turn mentored his own cohort of future illustrious scientists, many of them likewise physicians. Among their numerous students were Ernst Felix Hoppe-Seyler, Friedrich Daniel Recklinghausen, Adolf Kussmaul, Ivan Pavlov, Adolf Fick, William Welch, Max Planck, Otto Frank, A. A. Michelson, Eugene Dubois, Robert Koch, and Sigmund Freud.

As highlighted elsewhere in this volume, the pivotal role of influential mentoring in inspiring and nurturing successful medical researchers is certainly no less important today. There are numerous illustrations of scientific communities in which explosive productivity has resulted from favorable conditions for research coupled with a rich network of mentoring across generations. A relatively recent example in the United States is the extraordinary incubator of talent that was built in the intramural research program of the National Institutes of Health in the post–World War II decades.

Yet it was a contemporary Frenchman, without any of the institutional resources of the mid-nineteenth-century German physician-scientists, who is today widely considered to be the founder of modern experimental medicine. Claude Bernard (1813–1878), a failed winegrower's son, a rejected playwright, and a struggling student, managed to graduate from the medical school of the University of Paris. He had the good fortune to intern at the Hôtel-Dieu under François Magendie, a physician whose bold approach to physiological experimentation captivated Bernard. Like his compatriot physiologists, Bernard did his research under primitive conditions, working in a damp cellar with virtually no equipment and only a few surgical instruments to perform animal vivisection. In fact he did not even have a real laboratory until Emperor Napoleon III built him one after he had become the celebrated chair of physiology at the Sorbonne, well after his most important contributions had been completed. Among these were groundbreaking studies of the physiology of digestion and the discovery of vasomotor nerves.

Bernard was guided by the concept of absolute determinism, which dictated that a phenomenon will not occur differently given the same conditions, and thus variations must be the result of some intervention that modifies the phenomenon. He completely rejected teleological explanations. While he acknowledged the importance of anatomy, he insisted that physiological processes were the result of physicochemical causes, and therefore physiology was not just "anatomy in motion." This led to Bernard's conceptual leap of a *milieu intérieur*, the unifying model that higher organisms have developed mechanisms to maintain the conditions of their tissues constant even as the conditions of the environment change.

This was the precursor of Walter Cannon's theory of homeostasis in the twentieth century.

But Bernard's greatest contribution was the "experimental method," in which he repudiated his mentor Magendie's empiricism. As described in his masterwork, *An Introduction to the Study of Experimental Medicine*, the experimental method involves the linked sequence of observation, hypothesis, and experiment to test the hypothesis; the results of experiments then themselves become new observations, which in turn lead to another hypothesis and experiment, and so forth. Bernard's articulation of the testing of hypotheses remains the cornerstone of experimental biomedical research today. Though a physician himself, Bernard shunned the kind of clinical medicine practiced by "observing physicians." He said: "I consider the hospital the antechamber of medicine. It is the first place where the physician makes his observations, but the laboratory is the temple of the science of medicine." Claude Bernard, the peerless experimentalist and thinker, left no research school and was a brilliant flash in this relatively bleak period of French medical history (Conti 2001).

Discovery of Cells and Germs

The great German tradition of university-based medical research institutes spawned Rudolf Virchow (Reese 1998). Virchow's transformative studies in pathophysiology were firmly anchored in his earlier career experience as a practicing military physician and surgeon at the famous Charité Hospital in Berlin. His monumental body of work launched the era of the cellular basis of disease. Cell theory, the foundation of modern biology, was formulated only a few years earlier. The German botanist Matthias Schleiden (1804–1881) had demonstrated that cells were the basic, self-reproducing units of plants, and the physician Schwann, an earlier student of Müller, had shown the same in animal tissues. Now Virchow proposed that abnormal but likewise self-reproducing cells also explained pathology: "omnis cellula e cellula" (all cells from cells).

Although Virchow's doctrine of the cellular basis of disease set the stage for the microbiological revolution ignited by Pasteur and Koch, Virchow himself could not accept the germ theory of disease, which posited that human disease could be caused not only by a breakdown of order within the cells of the body but also by the invasion of the body from the outside by foreign cells.

While the centuries of advances in medicine up to the time of Pasteur contributed to an ever-accelerating expansion of basic information about health and disease, virtually none of this knowledge could be considered to have had a direct impact on the prevention or treatment of human disease.

(The one notable exception might be vaccine development. Even this, however, was a largely empirical advance, the scientific underpinnings of which were not at all understood.) As a result of its failure to cure any disease, the medical profession was not held in high esteem prior to the mid-nineteenth century. In Molière's play *Le Malade Imaginaire*, the brother of the hypochondriac title character notes about the ineffective, pompous doctors gathered around him: "And what are they really doing? I'll tell you. They're quoting from the collected novels, short stories, and fairy tales of that fertile old hack called Medicine. Visit your local bookshop, look under 'F' for Fiction.... [D]reams, doctors are peddlers of dreams." And Benjamin Franklin remarked that "God heals and the doctor takes the fee."

The germ theory for the first time identified causation of disease. Ironically, while most of the great contributions to medical knowledge up to this time had been made by physicians, the microbiological discoveries that led directly and in rapid succession to dramatic new cures were made by a nonphysician. Louis Pasteur (1822–1895) was trained as a chemist, and his early work on control of the fermentation process was motivated largely by industrial, not medical, progress. But after his election to the French Academy of Medicine in 1873 by but a single vote, he devoted the rest of his life to applying his germ theory to the eradication of disease.

It is important at this point to remark that, although this chapter focuses on the irreplaceable and vital role of physicians in medical research throughout history, the contributions of nonphysician scientists have been and continue to be at least as important. Even during this early period of the rise of science in medicine, investigators from a wide variety of nonmedical backgrounds made discoveries that were to have an incalculable impact on today's practice of medicine. In addition to the chemist Pasteur, some of these early nonphysician giants included the physicist Wilhelm Conrad Roentgen (1845–1923), the discoverer of X ray; the botanist Dmitri Ivanovsky (1864–1920), the discoverer of viruses; the priest and physics teacher Gregor Mendel (1822–1884), the "father of genetics"; and the zoologist Elie Metchnikoff (1845–1916), who pioneered cellular immunity with the discovery of phagocytes. Later in the twentieth century and beyond, the vital engagement of nonphysicians in the medical research enterprise would continue to increase.

Pasteur and Robert Koch (1843–1910) came to pioneer the germ theory of disease from strikingly different backgrounds and perspectives (Ullman 2007). Pasteur was a physical scientist who instinctively pursued his work into the arena of medicine through his quest for not only fundamental understanding but also practical application of his research. He repeatedly asserted that there are not two forms of science—pure and applied—but only science and the application of science. (The imperative for a cooperative rather than an opposing relationship between research for the sake of understanding and research for the sake of application is brilliantly developed in Donald Stokes's book *Pasteur's Quadrant,* titled in tribute to Pasteur's work [Stokes 1997].) By the time Pasteur plunged into infectious diseases research, he was already an accomplished scientist, having made important contributions to understanding the crystal structure of organic molecules, discovered that microorganisms participate in fermentation, and developed the process of sterilization subsequently called "pasteurization."

Koch, twenty years his junior, was still in medical school at the University of Göttingen in 1865 when the silkworm industry of Europe was decimated by what Pasteur was to prove to be microbial pathogens. After his medical studies, Koch served as a military physician in the Franco-Prussian War in 1871 and then became a country doctor with an extensive clinical practice. Anthrax is a highly contagious disease that commonly affected livestock, creating agricultural disasters, and sometimes also infected humans. During his free time Koch constructed a primitive laboratory at home and, using a microscope that was a birthday present from his wife, began to identify consistently the same rod-shaped structures in blood from sheep that had died from anthrax. Koch later discovered and described the life cycle of the anthrax bacillus, even as Pasteur was working in France on an anthrax vaccine. Thus Koch and Pasteur independently performed research on anthrax, eventually developing an intense rivalry that was undoubtedly fueled by nationalistic passions in the aftermath of the Franco-Prussian War. Their combined body of work, however, provided experimental evidence that the anthrax bacillus is responsible for the disease, thereby establishing the germ theory. As Pasteur and Koch gained great fame, it was not long before they and their students identified the causes of many other infectious diseases in rapid succession, including history's great public health scourges such as tuberculosis, cholera, diphtheria, typhoid, and syphilis.

In addition to their studies of the causation of individual diseases of humans and animals, Pasteur and Koch were also the architects of the concepts of "virulence" and "pathogenicity." Pasteur recognized that the capacities of microorganisms to cause disease were not an absolute property but could be altered by a variety of conditions. Koch in turn developed his time-honored postulates that must be met to prove causation of any infectious disease: (1) an organism must be found in every case of the disease,

(2) the organism must be isolated and grown in pure culture, (3) the cultured organism must produce the same disease when introduced into a healthy animal, and (4) the same organism must be recovered again from the inoculated experimental animal that has developed the disease.

The Evolving Role of the Physician as Scientist during the Early Twentieth Century

By the end of the nineteenth century, the dramatic rise of science and research in medicine had begun to change profoundly the way medicine was taught in the great European medical schools. Science had become integral to the education of medical students. These schools began to create true preclinical curricula and appointed full-time basic scientists to teach subjects such as anatomy, pathology, physiology, and later biochemistry, bacteriology, and pharmacology. Some leading American medical schools, including Johns Hopkins, Harvard, and the University of Pennsylvania, whose faculty had trained in Europe, followed suit. But it was not until the 1910 publication of the Carnegie Foundation's transformative report by Abraham Flexner, *Medical Education in the United States and Canada*, that American medical schools began to require uniformly the incorporation of rigorous courses in the medical sciences and even the prerequisite of a minimum of two years of undergraduate studies primarily devoted to basic science. By the end of the first decade of the twentieth century, the United States had surpassed Germany in producing the world's largest share of medical discoveries. Therefore this section primarily follows the evolution of physicians in medical research in North America during the twentieth century as the prototype of changes elsewhere in the world.

In the post–Flexner Report years PhD scientists began to replace physicians on the faculties of preclinical departments. They also increasingly provided postgraduate research training opportunities for medical school graduates who were interested in investigative careers. At least until World War II, however, the research conducted in these preclinical departments, even by the ever-increasing number of PhDs, was firmly rooted in clinical questions based on the study of patients. Indeed research laboratories were located almost invariably in hospitals. The close proximity of laboratories and hospital wards allowed medical students to observe continuously the daily activities of their professors, coming and going between bedside and bench, and often transmitting to them a contagious passion for medical research.

As Ludmerer has noted, the allure of research to medical students in the first half of the twentieth century was enhanced by the conspicuous disdain of researchers for commercialism and their lack of interest in personal financial reward (Ludmerer 1999). In part this reflected the early-twentieth-century tension between the traditionally unscientific practice of medicine and the reductionist, experimentalist philosophy of scientific research. Sinclair Lewis's *Arrowsmith*, published in 1925, traces the fictional education and career of the title character, an idealistic young physician who is repeatedly tempted by the comforts, social status, wealth, and power of private practice and corporate medicine. He is ultimately guided by his mentor, Max Gottlieb (not without point depicted as an immigrant German Jewish scientist), who embodies the stereotype of the incorruptible, altruistic, dispassionate researcher (Fangerau 2006). Gottlieb tells Arrowsmith: "There is one thing I keep always pure: the religion of a scientist.... He speaks no meaner of the ridiculous faith-healers and chiropractors than he does of the doctors that want to snatch our science before it is tested and rush around hoping they heal people. He is the only real revolutionary, the authentic scientist, because he alone knows how liddle [sic] he knows" (Lewis 1925).

The increasing glamour of medical research in the first half of the twentieth century was heightened by the introduction of dramatic therapeutic advances. The battlefields of the two world wars proved to be laboratories for the treatment of infectious diseases. Following the extraordinary burst of discoveries of microorganisms responsible for specific infectious diseases by the "microbe hunters" of the last two decades of the nineteenth century, effective immunization was developed against tetanus by the British physician Almroth Wright (1861–1947), and antitoxin against tetanus was produced by two other physicians, Koch's pupil Kitasato Shibasaburo (1853–1931) and Emil Adolf von Behring (1854–1917). Tetanus antitoxin was given to wounded soldiers in World War I, while tetanus immunization was administered to all military personnel sent abroad.

The work of the German physician-scientist Paul Ehrlich (1854–1915) was stimulated by the idea that the structures of chemicals were the keys to the potential actions of biologically active compounds on microbes. He thus pioneered the concept of chemotherapy. He developed the first antibiotic drug in modern medicine, albeit not the "magic bullet" he had hoped for, when he tested hundreds of arsenical compounds against the causative bacterium of syphilis and found that "compound number 606" was effective. Ehrlich subsequently discovered the bacteriostatic activity of sulfa drugs against streptococci, thus realizing Semmelweis's dream of conquering puerperal fever in mothers after childbirth. While the relationship between the pharmaceutical industry and academic pharmacology was troubled by the conflict between the profit motive and scientific freedom from its earliest days, Ehrlich's Frankfurt Institute research laboratories were able to develop particularly constructive ties with pharmaceutical companies.

The story of the serendipitous discovery of penicillin in 1928 by the Scottish bacteriologist and physician Alexander Fleming (1881–1955) is the stuff of legend. Fittingly it was Pasteur, the founder of germ theory, who had remarked seventy-five years earlier that "in the field of observation, chance favors only the prepared mind." Returning from vacation to his laboratory at St. Mary's Hospital in London, Fleming found that a petri dish of cultured staphylococci he had left on the bench was contaminated with a mold, but that remarkably the bacteria were not growing immediately around the mold. (This was not the only "serendipitous" observation the modest Fleming made during his career.) It was not until a decade later that an Australian physician-scientist, Howard Florey, and his team at Oxford purified penicillin from the mold. Successfully tested by Florey on wounded soldiers in North Africa in 1943, penicillin was rushed into mass production by British pharmaceutical companies and had become available to treat all military personnel by D-day. Also during World War II the Russian immigrant microbiologist Selman Waksman (1888–1973) discovered the first effective treatment for tuberculosis: streptomycin.

In addition to these antimicrobial treatments, by the middle of the war a variety of other therapeutic agents had entered medical practice, including heparin, insulin, and vitamins. By mid-century the long-awaited therapeutic revolution was in full bloom.

Postwar Boom in Medical Research: The Molecular Era

The course of World War II immensely increased the public's respect for science, particularly in the United States. Technology was widely viewed as the key to winning the war. In 1944 President Franklin D. Roosevelt commissioned a report from Vannevar Bush, his influential director of the wartime Office of Scientific Research and Development, on how the nation might build on its investment in scientific research in the peacetime years that lay ahead. In *Science, the Endless Frontier*, Bush argued passionately for continued growth of federal support for scientific research, and succeeded in securing the marriage between science and government for the decades to come. No other government agency reaped the sustained benefit from the enormous postwar expansion in federal support for research more than the National Institutes of Health. From its status prior to the war as a small agency that supported mostly in-house (intramural) medical research, the NIH now blossomed into a national biomedical research engine with a vast extramural research enterprise to complement its thriving intramural program. Its budget grew 150-fold between 1945 and 1961, reaching $1 billion by the late 1960s and almost $30 billion by the first decade of the twenty-first century. Over the course of the second half of the twentieth century, strong bipartisan support in Congress, postwar prosperity, rising expectations for longevity and good health, the growing influence of constituency groups, and the public's faith in medical research drove and sustained support for the NIH that outstripped government funding for other sciences. Capital financing of buildings and equipment for medical research was catalyzed by the Health Research Facilities Construction Act of 1956. In addition, the power of advocacy for disease-targeted research reached new heights in the early 1950s with the development and mostly successful deployment of polio vaccines through the support of the March of Dimes. Philanthropy, which had been the mainstay of medical research support prior to the war, continued to fuel this postwar golden age for medical research.

The enormous expansion of government support for biomedical research in the United States was later mirrored on a more modest scale in other countries, for example, by the Medical Research Council (MRC) in the United Kingdom and the Institut National de la Santé et de la Recherche Médicale (INSERM) in France.

Two important and powerful postwar currents changed the focus of medical investigation to basic research and introduced PhD scientists to the medical research enterprise in unprecedented numbers. First, medical research was becoming increasingly reductionist, concentrating more and more on using physical and chemical analyses to elucidate life processes at a subcellular and molecular level. The discovery of the double helix structure of DNA by Watson and Crick in 1953 was an important catalyst in this movement. Second, medical research continued to follow the postwar aphorism of Vannevar Bush, which affirmed the primacy of pure basic research without the necessary consideration of any practical ends. Nonphysician scientists recognized the burgeoning opportunities created by the NIH and increasingly established their laboratories in clinical departments of medical schools. Between 1981 and 1999 the number of PhD faculty who had their primary appointments in clinical departments grew 115 percent—from 5,657 to 12,141—higher than the growth rates for PhDs in basic science departments or even MDs in clinical departments (Fang and Meyer 2003).

By the end of the twentieth century, the molecular era was firmly entrenched. Basic biomedical research was increasingly dominated by nonphysician scientists. There was a growing separation between those who were conducting primarily laboratory research (including those with MD degrees) and those who were practicing clinical medicine. Indeed an increasing language and cultural barrier was actually developing between laboratory scientists and clinicians. New biomedical laboratory research buildings in academic medical centers were being constructed at sites physically removed from the hospitals. Ludmerer has referred to this as "an architectural embodiment of the shift of clinical investigation from a patient focus to a laboratory focus" (Ludmerer 1999). And those remaining physicians who were committed to research careers were increasingly turning away from basic science to pursue patient-oriented research, including clinical trials, epidemiology, and the new areas of health services, outcomes, and medical informatics research.

So the evolving role of physicians in medical research during the twentieth century can be summarized as follows. From the 1890s to the 1930s, laboratory research conducted by physicians was tightly linked to medical practice and public health. Basic research was inspired by clinical observations ("bedside-to-bench" research). It was greatly facilitated by the development of new instruments (X ray, electrocardiograph) and new methods in clinical chemistry to permit measurements in patients, as well as the creation of specialized wards and laboratories within hospitals. From the 1930s to World War II, public adulation grew for basic biomedical scientists, who were still mostly physicians. Yet these investigators, supported mainly by philanthropy, were now increasingly pursuing research into basic biological processes that became progressively detached from direct clinical relevance. PhD scientists were entering the medical research arena in increasing numbers.

World War II interrupted this trend, as medical researchers supported the war effort by returning to practical work. As soon as the war ended, however, influenced by Vannevar Bush and the strong basic science orientation of a burgeoning NIH, fundamental research came to eclipse applied research in both support and prestige. PhD scientists now flooded the medical research enterprise. During this "golden age" of clinical research that lasted into the 1970s, many well-trained "triple threat" physicians, who pursued patient care, teaching, and research simultaneously (though with an increasingly predominant commitment to research) were able to remain competitive with PhD scientists, who were not burdened by the distraction of patient care responsibilities.

By the 1970s there was mounting pressure from Congress for the NIH to pursue medical research that would result in practical payoff for patient care, as well as increasing pressure from patient advocacy groups seeking the conquest of specific diseases. An important catalyst for this reorientation was the Bayh-Dole (University Small Business Patent Procedures) Act of 1980, which greatly facilitated the ability of universities to patent and license the products of their federally financed research activities. For the first time universities, academic medical centers, and even their individual faculty members could profit from market transfer of their research. Institutional "tech transfer" offices boomed. (While well intentioned, the Bayh-Dole Act has subsequently seen the potential for perverse incentives of profit motive trumping intellectual curiosity as the driver of medical research, as well as concern about proprietary interests discouraging the expeditious and open sharing of emerging discoveries.)

For the next two decades, scientists successfully repelled the repeated efforts of an increasingly impatient Congress and public to redirect them to more practical, clinically oriented research. Even in the face of the budgetary constraints of the early Reagan years, the NIH protected investigator-initiated fundamental investigation at the expense of patient-oriented research, such as clinical trials. As basic research and applied research became further polarized, physicians, who found it progressively more difficult to keep up with their basic scientist colleagues, began to abandon the former. Those who remained interested in research careers turned more and more to patient-oriented applied research, or to the rapidly growing fields of health services, outcomes, and epidemiology research. Others relinquished medical research altogether, ceding it to nonphysician scientists, and entered clinical practice and teaching careers.

Beginning in the 1980s, concerns about the physician-scientist as an "endangered species" began to be voiced (Wyngaarden 1979). With the explosion of molecular biology in the 1970s, clinical and basic biomedical research started to diverge dramatically. Urgent action was called for to revitalize clinically oriented research, including the 1994 report of the Institute of Medicine on overcoming the barriers to career paths for clinical research (Kelley; and Randolph 1994), the 1996 NIH committee chaired by David Nathan that proposed recommendations to address the perceived shortfall of clinical investigators (Nathan 1998; and see chapter 15 of this book), and the Association of American Medical Colleges' Task Forces on Clinical Research (Association of American Medical Colleges 2006b). The growing public perception that the enormous resources being poured into biomedical research are not resulting in commensurate gains in new treatments, diagnostics, and prevention of disease is now spurring action by medical research agencies in the United States and elsewhere in the world. In response to the ebbing movement of ideas and knowledge back and forth between bedside and bench, the term "translational research" was coined in the early 1990s (Butler 2008). In 2006, focused on translational research, the NIH attempted to catalyze a new culture of multidisciplinary team research by initiating funding for a consortium of Clinical and Translational Science Centers throughout the country. Similar initiatives are under way in other countries. A new era is dawning for the historically vital role of physicians in medical research.

2

Demographics of the Physician-Scientist Workforce

IMPACT OF AGE, GENDER, DEGREES, AND DEBT

Timothy J. Ley, MD

Physician-scientists are individuals who hold an MD degree and who perform medical research as their primary professional activity. Most physician-scientists have only the MD degree, but many have a second degree (e.g., PhD, MPH, MBA, JD). Although physician-scientists conduct scientific investigation along a broad range of topics, virtually all have been imprinted during their training by caring for patients. These clinical experiences shape the approaches of this unique group of investigators during their subsequent scientific careers.

A number of trends during the 1980s and 1990s suggested that this career pathway was in serious jeopardy (Gill 1984; Wyngaarden 1979; Zemlo et al. 2000; Weinberg, 2006; Schecter 1998; Rosenberg 1999; Goldstein and Brown 1997). More recent data have shown, however, that the number of physicians who perform research as their primary professional activity has been stable since the early 1980s (see figure 2.1) (Zemlo et al. 2000; Ley and Rosenberg 2005). This apparent stability nonetheless conceals a disturbing trend: the overall number of physicians in the United States has nearly doubled over the same period of time, so the proportion of physicians conducting research has decreased with respect to that larger pool. On the basis of these data, and assuming a career length of approximately twenty-five years, I would estimate that approximately five hundred to one thousand new physician-scientists per year are required to maintain the steady state. Between four to five hundred new MD-PhDs graduate from U.S. medical schools each year (G. Garrison, personal communication), and the

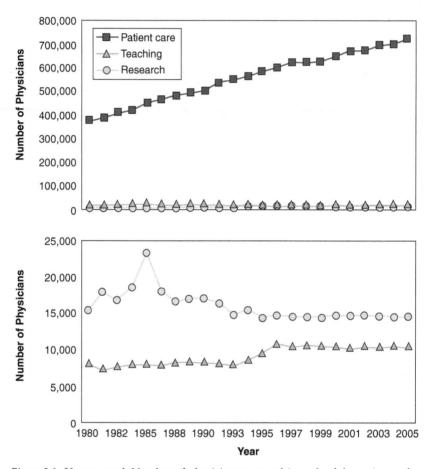

Figure 2.1. Upper panel: Number of physicians engaged in each of the major professional activities. Bottom panel: Expanded view of physicians whose primary research
activity is teaching and research. Source: American Medical Association.

majority of this group can be expected to become physician-scientists. The
rest of the pool must come from "late bloomer" MDs (discussed in chapter 10 by Kenneth Kaushansky), a tiny subset of the seventeen thousand
medical school graduates in the United States each year.

So is the physician-scientist career path really at serious risk? Several
protracted demographic trends suggest that it is.

Age

First, data from the National Institutes of Health clearly show that the
population of funded investigators is increasing in age. Figure 2.2a shows

that funded MD investigators (all investigators with NIH Research Project Grants [RPGs]) are the oldest of the degree holders, and that their average age has increased steadily since the mid-1980s. In 2006, 50 percent of MD RPG awardees were over the age of fifty (Zemlo et al. 2000; Ley and Rosenberg 2005). These trends are also true for PhDs, but as a group these investigators are significantly younger than funded MDs. Although it is not as striking as for MDs, the trend is also evident for MD-PhDs. A 2005 report from the National Academies has shown that the average age on receiving the first funded RO1/R29 (independent investigator) awards for PhDs is now forty-two years, for MDs forty-four years, and for MD-PhDs forty-three years (Council 2005). A variety of factors have contributed to this disturbing trend, but the consequence is clearly an aging population of investigators with relatively short independent research careers.

Gender

The second major demographic factor that will alter the composition of the physician-scientist workforce is gender (National Institutes of Health 2008a; Andrews 2002; Buckley et al. 2000; Guelich et al. 2002; Jagsi et al. 2006; Kaplan et al. 1996; Leboy 2008; Martinez et al. 2007; National Academy of Sciences 2006; Tesch et al. 1995). In 1981 only 25 percent of medical students were female. Now gender parity has been reached for medical school students (figure 2.2b). Why is this is an important demographic issue? As shown in figure 2.2c, medical school faculties in the United States display an enormous and persistent gender gap. Only about one-third of United States medical school faculty members are female, and this ratio has not changed substantially since the mid-1980s.

Furthermore, when academic rank is taken into consideration, there is gender parity at the instructor level, but significant drop-offs at each stage of promotion, so that only 17 percent of full professors are women. This pattern of persistent career attrition (the "leaky pipeline") has not changed substantially since the mid-1980s (National Institutes of Health 2008a; Andrews 2002; Buckley et al. 2000; Jagsi et al. 2006; Kaplan et al. 1996; Martinez et al. 2007). Unless this trend is altered, the physician-scientist workforce will likely decline. This represents the single most compelling challenge to the career pipeline; actions designed to address this issue must be a high priority for the NIH and academic medical center leaders (Ley and Hamilton 2008). Issues related to women physician-scientists are further discussed in depth in chapter 5 by Reshma Jagsi and Nancy Tarbell.

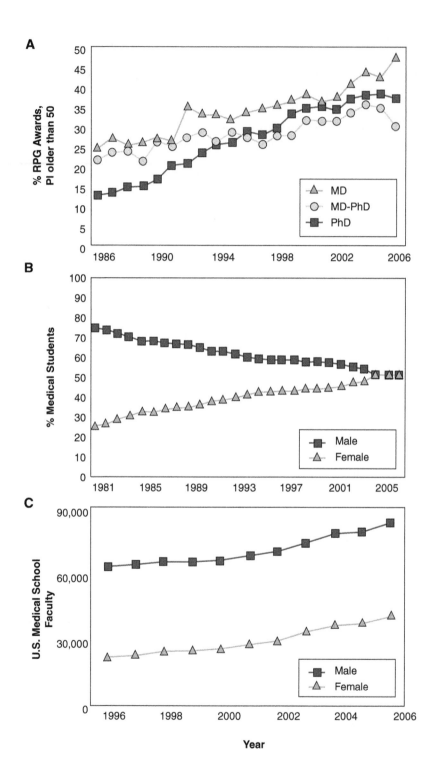

A

% RPG Awards, PI older than 50

- △ MD
- ◯ MD-PhD
- ■ PhD

B

% Medical Students

- ■ Male
- △ Female

C

U.S. Medical School Faculty

- ■ Male
- △ Female

Year

Degrees and Funding Success

A third demographic issue that could affect the stability of the physician-scientist career path is the success rate of these individuals in the NIH grant pool. Indeed, as discussed in detail in chapter 3 by David Korn and Stephen Heinig, a 2007 report by Dickler and colleagues suggested that there is a small but significant reduction in the success rates of investigators with an MD degree only for first-time RO1 grant applications, and also for RO1 renewals, compared to those with PhD or both MD and PhD degrees. Furthermore, these authors found that MD applicants were funded at lower rates for clinical than for nonclinical, basic research.

To look at these trends with a broader view of NIH grantees, I examined all research project grant (RPG) applications and success rates for MDs, MD-PhDs, and PhDs since 1986 (figure 2.3) (Ley and Rosenberg 2005). When all investigators are considered, it is clear that the vast majority of the increase in RPG applications (fueled by the period of doubling of the NIH budget between 1998 and 2003) has come from PhDs. The number of applications from MDs and MD-PhDs has also realized slow but steady growth over this period, and the number of MD applicants is still greater than that of MD-PhDs (who constitute only about 3 percent of medical school graduates). When success rates are considered for all RPG grants as a function of degree, it is clear that there is no major difference between the funding success rates of MDs, MD-PhDs, and PhDs. Although significant differences can exist from one year to the next, the overall trend is clearly that of equal success, regardless of the degree held. Finally, these trends remain true for both experienced and previously unfunded investigators; the success rates for all degree holders have become nearly identical.

These data are further validated when success rates for mentored K08 (career development) awards and for all RO1s are considered (figure 2.4). From 2003 to 2007, 94 percent (2,615 of 2,795) of K08 applicants were MDs and MD-PhDs; the success rates for MD-PhDs are slightly higher

---

Figure 2.2. Panel A: Percentage of NIH research project grant awards (RPGs) to principal investigators over the age of 50. Data are shown from the period 1986–2006 for the function of each degree type. For this and other figures, MDs include individuals with an MD degree alone as well as all individuals with an MD plus another professional degree other than the PhD. Similarly, MD-PhDs include all individuals with these two degrees plus any other professional degrees. Source: National Institutes of Health. Panel B: Percentage of matriculated medical students of each gender. Source: American Association of Medical Colleges. Panel C: Number of U.S. medical school faculty who are male and number who are female. Source: American Association of Medical Colleges.

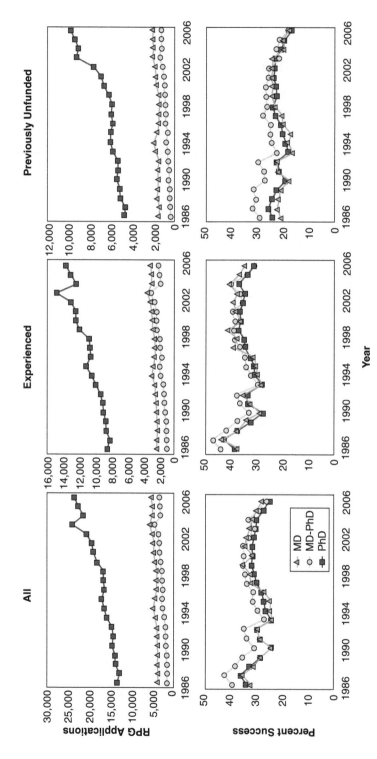

Figure 2.3. Number of NIH research project grant (RPG) applications and success rates for MDs, MD-PhDs, and PhDs as a function of experience. In the left-hand panels, all applications are considered. In the middle panels, individuals with previous funding from the NIH are considered. In the right-hand panels, only investigators who have previously been unfunded are considered. Source: National Institutes of Health.

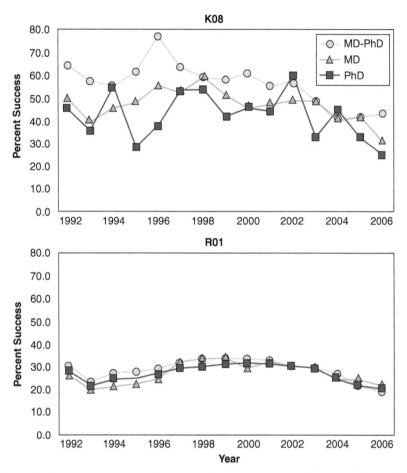

Figure 2.4. Percent success rates for KO8 applications and RO1 applications as a function of degree type and year. Note that MD-PhD applicants have tended to be more successful for KO8 applications, while all three degree types are virtually equally successful in the RO1 granting pool. Source: National Institutes of Health.

than those of MDs and PhDs for most years but not all. In the RO1 pool, the funding success rates for MDs, MD-PhDs, and PhDs have all been extremely similar since 1998, with a slow decline in success rates apparent from that year forward. In 2006, 997 RO1s were awarded to MDs and 694 to MD-PhDs. Therefore, 41 percent of the RO1s awarded to physician-scientists went to MD-PhDs, even though they account for only about 3 percent of medical school classes—again demonstrating the enormous enrichment of MD-PhDs in the physician-scientist workforce.

Debt

The fourth issue that could affect the long-term stability of the physician-scientist career path is that of medical school debt. As noted in several studies, the average debt for students attending private medical schools now exceeds $140,000, and is more than $80,000 for students attending public medical schools (Zemlo et al. 2000; Ley and Rosenberg 2005; Jolly 2005). In the late 1970s the average debt incurred in private medical schools was approximately equal to that of the average stipend of a PGY1 (first-year resident immediately out of medical school); the average debt incurred by students at publicly funded medical schools was less than half that (Ley and Rosenberg 2002). Since PGY1 stipends have increased at exactly the rate of inflation (Ley and Rosenberg 2005), medical school debt is now far greater than an average PGY1 stipend. Many believe that this growing debt factor could have a significant negative impact on the decision to become a physician-scientist.

To attempt to address this issue, the Association of American Medical Colleges (AAMC) has begun to ask graduating students about the influence of multiple factors on career choices, questions that were added to their graduating student questionnaire in 2005. During the period 2005–7, 7 percent of students felt that medical school debt was a strong influence on career choice, while 17 percent considered it a moderately important influence. Factors such as critical mentors play an even larger role, however, with 41 percent noting that a critical mentor was a strong influence on career choice, and 33 percent noting that it was a moderately important factor (Association of American Medical Colleges 2008a). Therefore, while medical school debt is an important issue, it is certainly not the only one that strongly influences the choice to seek a research career.

As medical school debt burdens mounted, the NIH initiated programs in 2002 that were designed to encourage recent medical school graduates to explore research careers during their fellowships (Ley and Rosenberg 2002; Nathan 2002). While performing approved types of clinically oriented research, physician-scientists in training could have up to $105,000 of their educational debt repaid (tax free). Although it is too early to assess the success of ongoing Loan Repayment Programs (LRPs), early data suggest that the pool of young physicians interested in research careers is much larger than had been previously thought (see figure 2.5). Approximately 2,000 individuals have applied for Loan Repayment Programs each year since 2004. Of these, approximately 500 are women with PhDs, and about 250 are men with PhDs. Remarkably, for MDs the number of male and female applicants is virtually identical (around 400 each year).

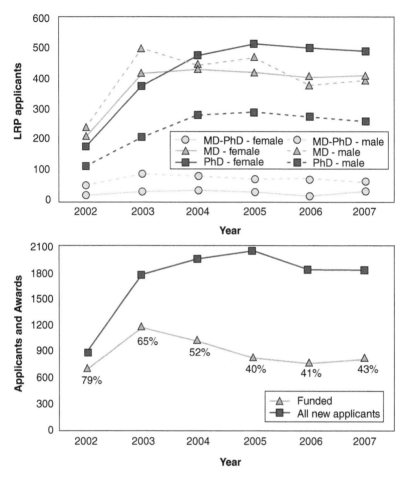

Figure 2.5. Number of applications and awards for NIH Loan Replacement Program Grants. The upper panel reveals the absolute number of LRP applicants since the inception of these programs in 2002. Applications are shown as a function of degree type and gender. The lower panel shows the total number of applicants and awards given from 2002 to 2007, including the percent success rates of applications shown on the line below the number of funded applications. Source: LRP Office.

MD-PhD applicants are fewer in number, since these individuals accrue a smaller medical school debt. As the number of applicants for LRPs has risen in recent years, the success rates have fallen somewhat, but leveled off in the 40 percent range (figure 2.5). Significantly, success rates for MD-PhDs are the highest of all LRP applicants (approximately 70 percent), but these applicants, as noted earlier, make up the smallest percentage of the total applicant pool. Success rates for MDs and PhDs are virtually equivalent. Although it is too early to know whether LRPs are influencing career decisions, the interest in this funding mechanism has been strong and sustained. LRPs are relieving the debt burden of more than three hundred new MD researchers annually, along with about seventy-five MD-PhDs. This may contribute significantly to the capture of "late bloomers" in research careers, and should help to stabilize the physician-scientist career pathway in the future.

Summary and Comments

The physician-scientist career path has been in steady state since the early 1990s, with no current evidence of significant attrition in the national workforce. Changing age and gender demographics, however, are creating potentially unstable conditions. Most important, now that gender equity has been reached for medical school students, gender-specific career attrition could have an enormous impact on the physician-scientist workforce in the future. Those with MD degrees only make up the largest pool from which to draw the physician-scientists of the future. Significantly, this group of individuals is *not* disadvantaged by competitive peer review in the NIH funding pool. Indeed, it is to be hoped that new interest in research careers has been stimulated by Loan Repayment Programs, which level the playing field for individuals with large medical school debts. Even if only a fraction of LRP holders successfully move their careers forward, this could have a significant impact on the physician-scientist workforce.

Questions for the Future

These demographic data raise a number of key questions that must be addressed by academic and government leaders in the years to come.

1. *How do we make a physician-scientist career path more sustainable for women?*
2. *Should MD-PhD programs be expanded? Is the talent pool expandable?* With debt levels rising, are MD-PhD programs beginning to attract applicants who are more interested in graduating from medical school debt free than in entering a research career?
3. *Should LRP programs be further expanded?* Is this applicant pool expandable without sacrifice of quality?

4. *Should KO8 funding be expanded to ensure the ultimate success of LRP grant holders and combined MD-PhD degree Medical Scientist Training Programs (MSTPs)?*
5. *Should first-time RO1 applicants receive preferential or extended funding periods for their first awards?*

The leaders of academic medicine should be encouraged to address these issues directly and to develop innovative, courageous, and visionary approaches that will succeed. Failure is unthinkable, because the stakes for biomedical research—and human health—are so high.

Acknowledgments

The author thanks all the people who helped assemble the data used in this report, including Robert Moore, Ernest Stalder, and Zhuohong Liu at the NIH Division of Information Services; Gwen Garrison, Jay Young-claus, and Hershel Alexander at AAMC; Derek Smart at the AMA; and Steve Boehler and Peggy Reed at the LRP Office. Lee Rosenberg and Stuart Kornfeld critically read the manuscript. This work was supported by the Alan A. and Edith L. Wolff Chair in Medicine at Washington University Medical School.

3

The Ecology of Physician-Scientists in Academic Medicine

David Korn, MD, and Stephen J. Heinig

Although few would deny that physician-scientists are essential to fulfilling the core missions of academic medicine—research, education, and patient care—or, indeed, that they are the only faculty who ideally embody all three of these missions, these investigators do not always see themselves as being thought essential or even welcomed within the maelstrom of the contemporary academic medical center. Yet since medical schools and teaching hospitals provide the unique breeding grounds for physician-scientists, whatever their later career paths, academic medicine is obliged to ensure that the national corps of physician-scientists is continually replenished and its robustness sustained. Not only is meeting this obligation critical to fulfilling the grand bargain struck by academic medicine with the American public in the aftermath of World War II—the promise that generous public support of basic biomedical research will lead to improvement of the health of the public—but it is also critical to the very survival of the American model of academic medicine.

Since the 1970s, concerns for the survival of the academic physician-scientist, and especially the translational and clinical scientist, have been articulated by eminent leaders of academic medicine. Hence the designation of these scientists as an "endangered species" (Wyngaarden 1979), the central theme of this book. In this and again in chapter 13 we provide a retrospective on a decade of studies and other initiatives undertaken by the Association of American Medical Colleges on behalf of physician-scientists generally and of clinical and translational investigators in particular.[1] As our analyses have shown, and the deliberations of our various task forces and advisory committees recognized, medical schools and teaching hospitals have undergone wrenching transformations since World War II, marked by enormous growth and increasing dependence on public funding for support of their research and clinical services missions. In recent years the social contract that has historically supported the ever-expanding roles of these institutions and taken a public stake in their continued vitality has become strained by new imperatives stimulated by historic federal fiscal deficits, unprecedented changes in the nation's demographics, projected physician shortages, and the looming insolvency of major entitlement programs. Contributing to that strain have been steadily tightening standards of public accountability accompanied by continuing revelations of faculty and institutional behaviors (for example, failure to disclose overly cozy relations with industry vendors and distortion or suppression of publication of industry-sponsored clinical trials results) that cumulatively erode public confidence and affront public trust. The future of academic medical centers as we know them will depend in large part on their ability to sustain public confidence in the integrity of academic medicine as a profession and in their ability to lead the nation in creating more effective, efficient, and equitable systems for delivering health care. This must be done while they continue to contribute through research to the health, prosperity, and security of the populace. Physician-scientists must play an essential role in responding to all aspects of these challenges.

In this chapter we provide an overview of the complex and dynamic ecology of academic medical centers and describe some of the antecedents that helped shape the AAMC's agenda-setting and policy analyses to support physician-scientists and clinical and translational research. We summarize our own analyses of stagnation in the numbers of new physician-scientists applying annually for National Institutes of Health (NIH) research project (R01) grants.

1. The Association of American Medical Colleges is a not-for-profit association representing all 131 accredited U.S. and 17 accredited Canadian medical schools; nearly 400 major teaching hospitals and health systems, including 68 Department of Veterans Affairs medical centers; and nearly 90 academic and scientific societies. Through these institutions and organizations the AAMC represents 125,000 faculty members, 70,000 medical students, and 104,000 resident physicians. For historical information about the AAMC, see Bowles and Dawson 2003.

The Ecology of Academic Clinical and Translational Research

Because of the unique role of medical schools and teaching hospitals in producing physician-scientists in the United States, understanding the ecology of academic medicine is critical to understanding the options available and the constraints faced by academic leadership and policymakers in training and sustaining physician translational and clinical scientists. As shown in figure 3.1, the academic medical enterprise has grown approximately 150-fold since the early 1960s as measured in total nominal expenditures. Primarily in response to the enactment in 1965 of Medicare and Medicaid legislation, which transformed much of the charity care on which the bulk of clinical education and training was then based into a revenue-generating business line, the patient care mission of academic medicine grew enormously and disproportionately, and all three missions of academic clinical departments became increasingly dependent on revenues from clinical services. These revenues have since the late 1980s accounted for about 50 percent of aggregate annual medical school expenditures (figure 3.2). To accommodate the demands of the relentlessly expanding health care delivery systems, the numbers of full-time faculty in the clinical departments increased nearly fifteen-fold, an expansion that was marked by a flowering of new faculty titles and lines, all of them non–tenure accruing and largely self-supporting. As we address later in this chapter, these changes in the terms and conditions of full-time faculty appointment in the clinical disciplines have had a profound impact on clinical scholarship, research, and training, on undergraduate clinical education, and on the culture of academic medicine.

In the 1960s funding from research and research support, mainly from the NIH, constituted nearly 55 percent of aggregate medical school expenditures (and clinical revenues less than 5 percent); total numbers of full-time faculty in the basic science and clinical departments were, respectively, about four thousand and seven thousand. In spite of nearly continuous real growth in the NIH budget averaging 3.5 percent per annum during this time span, with doubling of the budget on average every eight or nine years (Korn et al. 2002), and an approximately fivefold growth in number of basic science faculty, research funding as a share of total medical school expenditures has hovered around 20 percent for over two decades.

Throughout the same interval it is noteworthy that the total number of MD graduates only doubled (Association of American Medical Colleges 2006a), and the average share of total expenditures contributed by

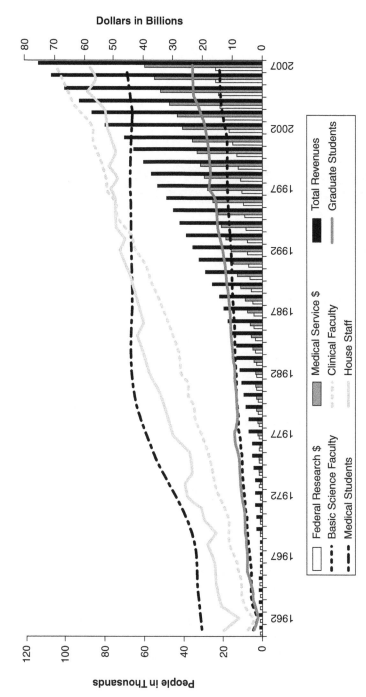

Figure 3.1. Growth in medical school faculty, students, and revenue, FY 1961–FY 2007. Figure prepared by Hershel Alexander, PhD, and Jonathan Lang, AAMC.

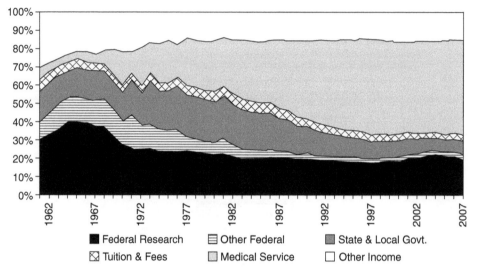

Figure 3.2. U.S. Medical school revenues and expenditures as a percent of total revenue, FY 1961–FY 2007. Figure prepared by Hershel Alexander, PhD, and Jonathan Lang, AAMC.

tuition income remained steady at less than 5 percent, while the numbers of graduate students, postdoctoral fellows, and residents increased many-fold. In an earlier publication (Korn 1998), one of us noted that these data might lead an observer reasonably to conclude that medical student education, the only mission unique to medical schools, had become a "distracting by-product" of academic medicine.

The NIH, of course, has been the predominant, albeit not exclusive, driver of the growth in research revenues to academic medical centers. Thus in 2006, the most recent year for which all data were available at the time of writing, medical schools and AAMC member teaching hospitals received 56 percent of the NIH's extramural budget for research and training (Fisher and Mays 2008). Other federal sources of clinical research funding include other Public Health Service agencies, the Departments of Defense and Energy, and, especially noteworthy, the Veterans Health Administration (VHA) of the Department of Veterans Affairs. The VHA maintains the nation's largest integrated health care delivery system, and 122 Veterans Affairs Medical Centers (VAMCs) are closely affiliated with 106 U.S. medical schools. These VA affiliates are largely staffed by medical school faculty and are substantially involved in undergraduate and graduate medical education as well as in medical research and training. Over the decades VAMCs have played an especially important role as "protected sites" for nurturing new physician-scientists.

The growth in national health expenditures and the costs of care, which rose at twice the rate of inflation until the 1990s, became increasingly restrained beginning in the 1980s and through the 1990s by more assertive intervention by federal, state, and private-sector payers and providers. Although "managed care" was often indicted as the principal driver of cost containment in academic medical centers in the later 1980s and 1990s, other private and governmental payers for health care were likewise seeking ways to contain growth in hospital and other health costs and expenditures. In this new economy, academic medical centers had to respond to competitive pressures from other health providers, especially nonacademic providers that did not have to bear the costs of education, research, or the provision of special high-intensity regional services (such as burn centers). As a result, there was relentless pressure on the then common practices of cross-subsidizing research and education, and especially clinical scholarship, with overages from clinical services, as well as providing "free access" to costly core facilities and instrumentation. Clinical faculty were increasingly pressured to devote more effort to providing services at the cost of previously protected time for research and training, and eventually for medical student education. In trying to adapt to the new economic circumstances of health care delivery, many academically affiliated hospitals and health systems were corporately restructured or transferred to new ownership, which in a number of cases sharply constrained opportunities to conduct clinical research, especially hypothesis-driven research and training (Heinig et al. 1999).

Growth of the academic clinical enterprise has resulted in faculty practice plan income becoming the largest single source of revenue for medical schools (figure 3.3a), particularly for private schools, followed by federal and nonfederal support for research. Among "research-intensive" institutions (that is, the twenty ranked highest in receipt of NIH awards; figure 3.3b), sponsored research support provides about 43 percent of annual expenditures in public medical schools and 33 percent in private schools. Of this support, federal sources, predominantly the NIH, account for 70 percent of the total in both public and private schools. As the figures show, what may be labeled institutional "hard money" provides only about 10 percent of total annual expenditures. Moreover, all major sources of funding are obligated to specific commitments. Even such sources as gifts and endowment income or state funding (primarily but not exclusively available to public schools) are typically obligated for specific purposes that are legally binding. Tuition, though costly and a target of growing public concern, provides a very small share of revenues and contributes only modestly toward compensating total educational expenses

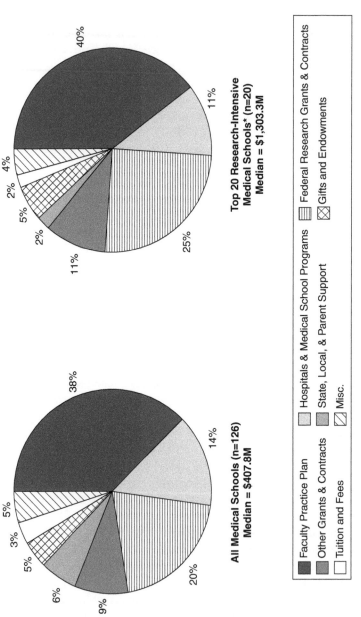

All Medical Schools (n=126)
Median = $407.8M

38%
14%
20%
9%
6%
5%
3%
5%

Top 20 Research-Intensive
Medical Schools* (n=20)
Median = $1,303.3M

40%
11%
25%
11%
2%
5%
2%
4%

- Faculty Practice Plan
- Hospitals & Medical School Programs
- Federal Research Grants & Contracts
- Other Grants & Contracts
- State, Local, & Parent Support
- Gifts and Endowments
- Tuition and Fees
- Misc.

Figure 3.3a. Total medical school revenue by source, FY 2007. Figure prepared by Hershel Alexander, PhD, and Jonathan Lang, AAMC.

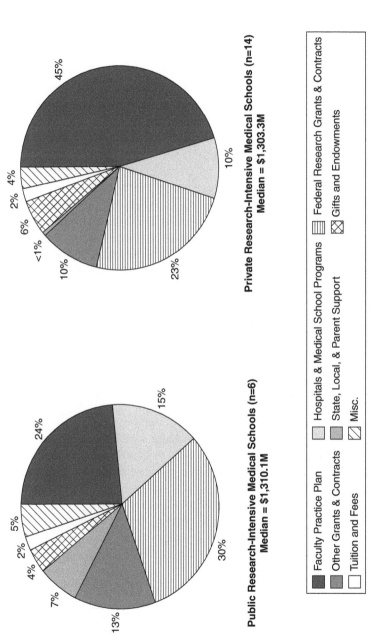

Public Research-Intensive Medical Schools (n=6)
Median = $1,310.1M

Private Research-Intensive Medical Schools (n=14)
Median = $1,303.3M

Faculty Practice Plan · Hospitals & Medical School Programs · Federal Research Grants & Contracts · Other Grants & Contracts · State, Local, & Parent Support · Gifts and Endowments · Tuition and Fees · Misc.

Figure 3.3b. Total medical school revenue by source, FY 2007: top 20 research-intensive medical schools. Figure prepared by Hershel Alexander, PhD, and Jonathan Lang, AAMC.

(Jones and Korn 1997). Yet tuition income remains one of the major sources of discretionary funding available to the institution, a reason AAMC has consistently but unsuccessfully opposed arbitrary caps on tuition reimbursements under federal training programs.

From these data two important considerations must be kept in mind regarding the current and future sustainability of academic medical centers. First, for two generations the system has equilibrated revenues and investments in expectation of steady and continuous growth in public support, and a "chronic and growing gap [has developed] between academic medicine's seemingly insatiable demand for total resources and the supply of resources that society is willing to provide" (Korn 1998). Second, the academic medical system—particularly research—is extraordinarily dependent on "soft" money. In consequence, the leadership of academic medical centers must make long-term commitments to capital expenditures (buildings, instrumentation, and so on) and personnel (hiring of staff, faculty recruitment, tenure, advancement and promotion, and the like) on the basis of anticipated revenues from clinical services, federal grants, and other external sources that are now capriciously subject to change. Planning and operations of academic medical centers are therefore extremely sensitive to tremors such as changes in risk or availability of funding for the research, teaching, and patient care missions, and arguably, above all, changes in public confidence and trust in the proposition that all of the missions of academic medicine are being conducted for the benefit of the public.

Endangered Species

Wyngaarden's initial observation of the decline of clinical investigation and physician-investigators in the United States led him to declare these scientists an "endangered species," but ironically, little of Wyngaarden's analysis actually considered the environmental context that was contributing to their endangerment (Wyngaarden 1979). Subsequent analyses were often even less considerate of underlying factors. Ahrens, at Rockefeller University, undertook perhaps the most methodical effort to evaluate rigorously what he considered a "crisis" in clinical research and attempted to distinguish at least some of the institutional and organizational drivers of decline (Ahrens 1992). Devising a specific seven-tiered definition of "clinical research," Ahrens measured the scope of activities in each tier using bibliometric and other indicators of scientific productivity among medical school faculty and other investigators. He concluded that hypothesis-testing, patient-oriented research (POR) was declining relative to less valued clinical reports and case studies and found these trends more pronounced among harried junior and associate clinical faculty than among more senior, better-established faculty. Ahrens identified the eroding environment within academic medical centers and, particularly, increased clinical service pressures on physician faculty as departmental and institutional subsidies for clinical investigation diminished as the leading culprit in this decline.

The most widely influential analysis, and the one that most effectively advanced reform after nearly two decades of hand-wringing, focused not on academic medical centers but on the NIH (Nathan 1998). Established by NIH director Harold Varmus in 1997 and led by David Nathan, president of the Dana-Farber Cancer Institute (and a contributor to this volume), the NIH Advisory Committee on Clinical Research largely substantiated concerns about challenges to training and support for clinical investigators while greatly moderating more stridently partisan concerns. The Nathan panel observed that the proportion of applications submitted by physicians for NIH research project grants had declined from 40 percent in 1972 to 25 percent in 1995, while the actual number of applications had nevertheless increased over that period. Although MDs and PhDs had approximately the same degree of success in receiving an award (an indication that the quality of the applications was comparable in peer review), the panel found that MDs with meritorious review scores who were declined a first award were less likely than PhDs to reapply. This finding, suggesting discouragement and preoccupation among physician-investigators, agreed with the view "in the trenches" reported by the NIH's clinical research ombudsman (Shulman 1996).

From a sample of NIH awards, the Nathan panel estimated that, notwithstanding proclamations to the contrary, 38 percent of the agency's extramurally funded research was "clinical" under the panel's definition, a proportion that the panel deemed reasonable. The panel concluded that NIH support for physician-led clinical investigation was more robust than many had believed, but that serious concerns about the vitality and future of clinical investigation were still justified, especially with regard to training and career development. The report arrived just as Congress decided to double appropriations for the NIH over the following five years, thereby enabling the agency to respond promptly by creating a suite of new K awards that included a mentored career development award program for new patient-oriented researchers, a mid-career POR award, an award to stimulate institutions to develop formal curricula for clinical research training, and a strengthened institutional training program in POR. The panel also made several recommendations that required and received congressional authorization. These included the establishment of an educational loan forgiveness program for new clinical investigators out of concern for the arguably career-directing role of the increasing indebtedness of graduating medical students (Jolly 2005), and expansion of the NIH's General Clinical Research Center (GCRC) award program.

Analyses of Physician-Scientists as First-Time Applicants for NIH Research Project Grants

To develop better empirical understanding of the scope of the clinician-scientist problem, and in response to many anecdotal reports by prominent faculty that well-qualified protégés were leaving the academic investigator track in discouragement, the AAMC undertook a historical assessment of physician-scientists' and clinical investigators' record of success relative to that of nonclinical scientists in applying for and receiving NIH R01 grants. While other studies had performed similar comparisons in particular years or over short time spans, we were especially interested in noting long-term historical trends to see how comparative success had changed over time. With the help of colleagues, we analyzed the number of individual first-time applicants for NIH research project grants (R01 awards) over the *entire* range of years recorded in the NIH's Consolidated Grant Applicant File (CGAF). There are other NIH and many private-sector research grant mechanisms, but the investigator-initiated, "curiosity-driven," hypothesis-testing R01 mechanism is widely regarded by NIH and the academic community as the quintessential award in establishing one's standing as an independent investigator and thereby advancing one's professional career.

The objectives, methods, and findings were provided in the original publication (Dickler et al. 2007). Briefly, the study addressed several questions, including: How has the number of first-time physician applicants for R01 grants varied over time? How did they fare, compared to PhD and MD-PhD applicants, in obtaining their first awards, reapplying for awards, and renewing awards? Have trends changed over time? Were applicants for R01s in human subjects research less or more successful than applicants not proposing research involving human subjects? Much of the data required for these analyses was available over a forty-year span (1964–2004). "First-time" applicants were defined as individuals applying for a first R01, regardless of whether they had applied for or received an earlier NIH award in another mechanism. We examined the records for all first-time applicants in each year represented in the CGAF.

The trends for first-time R01 applicants by degree are reproduced in figure 3.4. Although the number of MD-only physicians applying for a first

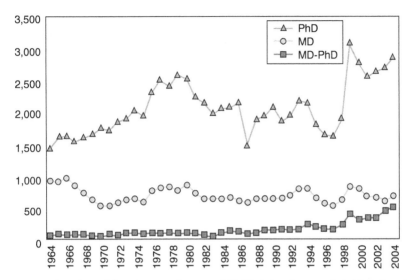

Figure 3.4. Number of first-time applicants to NIH R01s by degree, 1964–2004. Republished by permission of JAMA. Source: Dickler et al. 2007.

R01 fluctuated from year to year, it neither substantially increased nor decreased and, indeed, remained remarkably stable over the last generation. Through the whole range of the study (1964–2004), the net increase in annual number of first-time physician applicants (MD only plus MD-PhDs) was just 188 (from 1,012 to 1,200). In contrast, the number of first-time PhD applicants rose substantially between 1964 and 1980 and thereafter fluctuated considerably. It was this sharp decline *in the proportion* of physician-investigators in the NIH applicant and investigator pool that alarmed Wyngaarden and subsequent observers about physician-scientists' "failure to thrive."

Remarkably, even the doubling of the NIH budget from 1998 to 2003 did not spark an increase in the annual number of first-time physician (MD only) R01 applicants, although it did stimulate sharp increases in the annual number of first-time applicants with PhD and MD-PhD degrees (figure 3.5).

Although they remain a small proportion of the total, the number of first-time applicants with dual PhD and MD degrees increased steadily through the interval and by 2004 nearly equaled that of first-time MD-only applicants in the R01 pool. The NIH's Medical Scientist Training Program (MSTP), widely considered the "gold standard" of combined MD-PhD training, was launched in 1964 and has funded forty to forty-five programs

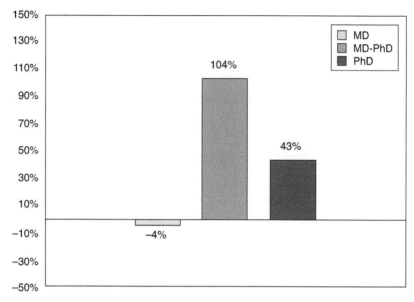

Figure 3.5. Percentage increase in number of first-time applicants for R01s by degree during the doubling of the NIH budget, 1998–2003. Figure by Di Fang, PhD, AAMC. Source: NIH CGAF.

for many years. There are, however, more than one hundred programs in U.S. medical schools, funded from diverse institutional and external sources. The remarkable growth in number of these programs reflects the consistent ability of MD-PhD graduates to compete successfully for NIH R01 (and other) grants; their growing attractiveness as department chairs and division heads, especially in the clinical disciplines; and, not least, the cachet that these programs bring to medical schools.

Among first-time R01 applicants, PhDs were only slightly more successful than MDs in winning an award (over the period studied, the mean success rate for MDs was 28 percent and that for PhDs was 31 percent); the difference was only modestly significant [p = .03]).

Among unsuccessful first-time applicants who reapply for an R01, 23 percent of physicians (MD only), 25 percent of PhDs, and 34 percent of MD-PhDs receive an R01 on a subsequent try. The difference for PhDs and MD-PhDs compared to MDs only is significant (p = <.001), and the difference is entirely due to the lower rate of reapplication by MD-only physicians, consistent with the finding of the Nathan panel (Nathan 1998). Similarly, among successful first-time applicants, PhDs and MD-PhDs were more likely to renew a first R01 or apply for a second R01 than were

MDs. It is important to recognize that the lower rate of reapplication for MDs was the major factor in their lower rate of receiving a second R01; that is, MD applicants for a second award were not competitively weaker than PhD applicants. MD-PhD investigators were most successful in receiving first and subsequent awards.

First-Time R01 Applicants in Human Subjects Research

The study also compared the effect on success of whether or not the PIs proposed to use "human subjects" in their initial application, as indicated by a checkbox first added to the R01 grant application form in 1980 and subsequently recorded in the CGAF.[2] The findings confirm the intuitive assumption that MDs are much more likely than PhDs to be involved in human subjects research (67 percent of MD-only applicants, 43 percent of MD-PhD applicants, and 39 percent of PhD only). Paradoxically, because PhDs so outnumber physicians in the applicant pool, 60 percent of all clinical applications are from PhDs, and this percentage is consistent across the years for which these data are available. In an earlier study Fang and Meyer (both at the AAMC) reported that clinical departments in U.S. medical schools experienced far higher rates of growth (1981–1999) in PhD faculty than did basic science departments, and indeed that the total PhD faculty in clinical departments outnumbers those in basic departments (Fang and Meyer 2003). Any considerations of the future clinical research workforce in academic medical centers must include training and support for PhD investigators.

Irrespective of degree, PIs applying for research projects involving human subjects were consistently and significantly less successful in their receipt and renewal of first-time R01 awards than their comparable colleagues proposing nonclinical research.

In a series of careful and informative studies, Kotchen and colleagues (Kotchen, Lindquist, Malik, and Ehrenfeld 2004; Kotchen et al. 2006; Martin, Lindquist, and Kotchen 2008) have confirmed the prevalent belief that human subjects research tends to be competitively disadvantaged in NIH

---

2. The human subjects checkbox in the grant application is, admittedly, an imperfect proxy for clinical research, as the check may also apply, for example, to research with human tissues or records but without direct interactions with human research subjects. As a result, this proxy would, if anything, overstate the number of R01s in clinical or patient-oriented research, and would predictably obfuscate differences between clinical and nonclinical research. That the differences observed are appreciable and significant underscores the very real differences in rates of success between human subjects and non–human subjects research. For further discussion, see methods section in Dickler et al. 2007.

peer review, but not for the reasons commonly opined, such as bias in the composition of study sections. Rather the perceived disadvantage can be nearly entirely explained by two factors: first, that a number of applications are administratively noted to have problems with the regulatory requirements that apply to human subjects research; and second, that in any pool of R01 applications reviewed in a given NIH cycle, the proportion of competing renewals in the basic sciences is significantly larger than that in the clinical sciences. Since the success rate of competing renewals is substantially higher than that of first-time applications, the overall success rate of the basic sciences subpool of applications is greater than that of the clinical sciences subpool.

To summarize, over the decades-long span of the available data, first-time applicants with only an MD degree are consistently less successful and less persistent than applicants with PhD or MD-PhD degrees. At every stage in the early life cycle of the R01 applicant—first award, subsequent application for renewal or for second award, and so on—MD-only investigators are less successful than their PhD and MD-PhD counterparts. The lower rate of success appears to be due primarily to the loss of MD-only investigators from the system, even after they receive a first R01 award. This "failure to thrive" of MD-only physician-investigators in the hotly competitive NIH R01 system is especially troubling in light of the remarkably expanding opportunities in biomedical research and the substantial real increases in NIH funding over the last several decades. The findings reflect, in our view, not an acute crisis but a chronic structural problem in academic medicine (Dickler et al. 2007).

A frustrating limitation of our (and others') analyses is the inability to determine whether MDs who drop out of the R01 cycle nonetheless remain engaged in research in academic medical centers, independent research institutes, industry, or elsewhere, or whether they abandon research entirely. The needed databases are simply not available (or accessible). AAMC staff are working with the MD-PhD section of the AAMC's professional development Group on Graduate Research, Education, and Training (GREAT) to develop and implement a Web-based system to track career outcomes for all U.S. MD-PhD program graduates (including but not limited to the NIH-sponsored MSTP).

The Supply of Junior Faculty Physician Clinical Investigators

To complement the R01 study, we examined with AAMC colleagues (Fang et al. 2007) recruitment of physician junior faculty in patient-oriented research in clinical departments. We surveyed 837 chairs of selected clinical departments at U.S. medical schools to determine the number of junior physician clinical investigators (MDs and MD-PhDs) in POR in these departments, the prevalence of open positions for such individuals, and success in filling these positions during the years 2002–2004. Sixty percent of the chairs surveyed completed the questionnaire. The survey frame was reasonably representative of the medical school population, and the distribution of the respondents adequately reflected the sample.

The results are shown in table 3.1. Most (68 percent) of the responding clinical departments reported having openings for junior physician-investigators in POR, totaling 2,097 over the three-year period. These data suggest that during the interval, approximately 3,500 such openings may have existed in U.S. allopathic medical schools. Notably, 52 percent of the departments with openings were not able to fill all positions, and 27 percent of all openings went unfilled. Although we cannot exclude that the large number of open positions may have been an artifact of the doubling of the NIH budget, we think it unlikely because overall growth in the total number of full-time faculty in clinical departments during the survey interval was only 8.9 percent (from 90,181 to 98,256 [Barzanksy and Etzel 2005]). Although the reported difficulty in recruitment was more severe in the less research intensive schools, even the most research intensive schools were unable to fill nearly one-fifth of their open positions. These findings

Table 3.1. Departments with open positions for MD assistant professors in patient-oriented research and positions that remained unfilled, by school research rank, 2002–2004

	Top 40 School		41–80 School		81–125 School		Total	
	#	(%)	#	(%)	#	(%)	#	(%)
Number of departments with openings (% of responding departments with openings)	154	(84%)	118	(69%)	66	(46%)	338	(68%)
Total number of openings (% of total openings by school category)	1310	(62%)	565	(27%)	222	(11%)	2097	(100%)
Number and (%) of departments with openings	69	(45%)	67	(57%)	40	(61%)	176	(52%)
Total number of openings (% of open positions that were not filled)	253	(19%)	215	(38%)	90	(41%)	558	(27%)

Source: Fang et al. 2007.

support the interpretation that insufficient numbers of junior physician clinical researchers are available to meet the current needs of the academic medical research agenda.

On the basis of these studies we conclude that ample quantitative evidence supports the research community's long-standing concerns about "the endangered species" and its reiterated warnings about the need for more clinical and translational researchers nationwide. Furthermore, we agree with Ahrens that the "eroding environment within academic medical centers" is a major factor contributing to the decline of clinical scholarship and to the difficulty of attracting young physicians into scientific careers, especially in patient-oriented research (Ahrens 1992).

Acknowledgments

The authors thank Hershel Alexander, PhD and Jonathan Lang of the AAMC for figures 3.1–3.3 and related information. Our colleague Di Fang, PhD, with the American Association of Colleges of Nursing, initiated together with David Korn the analyses of the NIH CGAF records and the survey of clinical department chairs recounted in this chapter.

4

Translational Research and the Physician-Scientist

Barry S. Coller, MD

Harnessing the power of the scientific method to improve health and alleviate suffering from disease is perhaps humankind's greatest achievement. We take for granted the connection between science and medicine, and so it is worth emphasizing that human observational science only began with Renaissance artists (Lucas 1955) and anatomists (Vesalius 1543) making detailed drawings of living and dead humans. Modern human experimental science really only began in 1865, when the French physiologist and physician Claude Bernard argued passionately that it was vital to develop human experimental science (Bernard 1927; Grande and Visscher 1967). It is probably no coincidence that Bernard wrote soon after Darwin published the *Origin of Species*, which marked the first public recognition that humans are members of the animal kingdom. Ironically, physicians were among those most opposed to medicine developing an empiric, experimental basis as opposed to applying the "well-established" principles of medical theory. The word "empiric" itself was originally used as a term of derision to describe physicians contemptible enough to rely on their

Supported in part by grant HL19278 from the National Heart, Lung and Blood Institute, and a Clinical and Translational Science Award (UL1 RR024143) from the National Center for Research Resources. The author discloses the following potential competing interest: Dr. Coller is an inventor of abciximab (Centocor), and in accord with federal law and the policies of the Mount Sinai School of Medicine he has a royalty interest in the VerifyNow assay system (Accumetrics). In addition he is a consultant to Accumetrics and is an inventor on a pending patent for a new antiplatelet compound.

own observations rather than well-accepted dogma (Trumble and Brown 2002)! Even Osler, probably the greatest observational medical scientist in history, who merged fastidious bedside examination with insightful and expert pathologic observations, was judged by those around him to be reluctant to embrace fully the experimental approaches developed primarily in Germany at the end of the nineteenth century (Bliss 1999; Cole 1949; Robinson 1957).

The establishment of the Rockefeller Institute for Medical Research Hospital in 1910 for the express purpose of making scientific discoveries to improve the therapy of disease could well be defined as the birth of translational research in the United States (Cole 1926). Rufus Cole, one of Osler's residents who left Johns Hopkins in pursuit of greater opportunities in experimental science, was named the first director of the Rockefeller Hospital. He successfully championed, against considerable resistance, the concept of the physician-scientist by insisting that the physicians at the Rockefeller Institute Hospital be provided with bench research space and resources. He looked to a time when the scientific base of medicine would be sufficiently rigorous to justify the creation of university departments of medicine on a par with departments in the natural sciences (Cole 1920). One of the great successes of his model and his astute recruitment was the 1944 discovery by Avery, MacLeod, and McCarty that DNA is the molecule that transmits hereditary information, a discovery that grew out of their clinical and bench research, as well as their medical care of more than one thousand patients with pneumococcal pneumonia (McCarty 1985; Dubos 1976).

The acceptance of medical school departments into the faculties of great universities and the further development of "university" hospitals have been the fulfillment of Cole's vision. Fueled by an enormous commitment of public funds through the National Institute of Health (NIH), this process reached its peak in the 1970s and 1980s. When seen against this sweep of history, the more recent trend for universities to distance themselves from their teaching hospitals financially and administratively, and in some cases to sell them outright to for-profit corporations, is an ominous sign for both the integration of medical research with medical care and the role of physician-scientist. The Clinical and Translational Science Award (CTSA) program instituted by the NIH in 2006 has the potential to reverse this trend at least partially, since it requires recipient institutions to organize and integrate their clinical and research structures so as to maximize their translational potential. It also has the potential to create a new discipline of clinical and translational science, with a cadre of outstanding trainees receiving advanced degrees in this new and evolving field. If successful, this augurs well for the future of the physician-scientist, but it will require broad commitment, creativity, a willingness to test new models, and substantial material and human resources.

In this chapter I first provide an operational definition of translational research and then consider the implications of that definition with regard to the importance of physician-scientists in achieving success in translational research. I then explore the essential elements in the training of physician-scientists, along with some of the cultural obstacles that have acted as impediments to careers in translational science. Finally, I offer some thoughts on potential strategies for developing a new cultural identity for physician-scientists.

What Is Translational Research and How Does It Fit into the Mission of the Academic Medical Center?

I began this chapter by emphasizing the extraordinary power of the scientific method to improve human health. From my vantage point, a major corollary of this principle is that research is not one of the missions of the academic health center—it is *the* mission. Many physician-scientists of my generation were influenced by the image of the academic medical center as a three-legged stool (figure 4.1), with research, patient care, and education all components of its mission. I believe that this image is seriously flawed and has had a deleterious impact on the structure and function of academic medical centers because it implies that research is an isolated, distinct enterprise separate from patient care and education. I believe we need a new image—a four-legged stool with a cushion (figure 4.2). In this model, research is the cushion that needs to be applied to all of the other components, maximizing their quality and effectiveness. Thus patient care, education, community service, and global health can all benefit from a commitment to apply the scientific method to achieve their goals. The last two elements are also inextricably linked to the attainment of social justice, and so it is important to emphasize to those searching for a career devoted to public service the enormous potential of scientific translational research to achieve social justice goals. For example, it has been estimated that the development by Merck of the drug ivermectin to treat onchocerciasis (river blindness) and Merck's decision to make the drug available for free has prevented more than six hundred thousand cases of blindness and returned millions of acres of arable land that had been abandoned back to productive farming (Amazigo et al. 2006).

The lack of a commitment to bring scientific methodology to medical education is most lamentable, resulting in our still lacking a solid base

The 3-Legged Stool

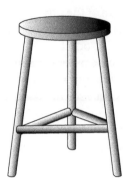

Research	Patient Care	Education

The 4-Legged Stool with Cushion

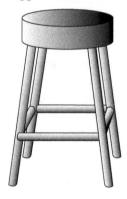

Research			
Patient Care	Education	Community Service	Global Health
		Social Justice	

Figure 4.1 and 4.2. Images of the missions of the academic health center. The three-legged stool (upper figure), composed of research, patient care, and education, must be updated (lower figure) to emphasize the importance of bringing the scientific method to improve all of the institution's missions. In addition, community service and global health have greater prominence and provide opportunities for connecting the medical mission to the attainment of social justice.

of empiric data on the effectiveness of different teaching methods. It is remarkable that there has been virtually no attempt to advance the field of medical education by conducting randomized controlled studies, the gold standard of the evidence-based medicine taught in medical school.

Against this background, I propose that translational research be defined as the application of the scientific method to address a health need. The spectrum is extremely broad, encompassing observational and experimental reductionist science, the science of clinical trial design, and the population-based sciences of epidemiology, community health, occupational health, health services research, and public health. Most important, since all of these disciplines can contribute to translational research, and there is extraordinary potential for synergism by integrating two or more of these disciplines in pursuit of a translational goal, each is worthy of equivalent academic recognition and support. Alvan Feinstein, a keen and thoughtful observer of academic medical centers, noted in 1999 that the academic respect received by an investigator was inversely proportional to the size of the object the investigator studied (Feinstein 1999). That perverse expression of fundamental values continues to haunt us, acting as a severe impediment to achieving our translational opportunities.

How Does Translational Research Differ from Basic Science Research?

Translational research differs from basic science discovery in both its goals and processes. Thus basic science research starts with the current scientific paradigm and systematically tests its validity by assessing whether predictions based on the paradigm are borne out by experiment. As long as the experiments are designed and conducted with rigor, new knowledge is obtained regardless of the results; the data either support the current paradigm or demonstrate that it needs to be modified or discarded.

In contrast, translational research starts with the articulation of a health need and then proceeds to search available scientific knowledge to identify insights or tools that can be harnessed to address the need. A multi-directional process between bench, bedside, and curbside then ensues to develop and refine the idea and convert it into a new drug, diagnostic approach, therapeutic device, or preventive strategy, ultimately resulting in a change in public health advice and/or medical practice. The final goal is not new knowledge but rather better health. Since one almost always lacks certain knowledge about the impact of any intervention in humans, and it is extremely challenging to design clinical studies to assess safety and efficacy unequivocally, the likelihood of success of a new approach is small. For example, only 10 to 20 percent of drugs that enter clinical trials go on to achieve regulatory approval (Wood 2006). Even failed clinical studies can, however, provide valuable information for the next attempt. It is extremely advantageous, therefore, for translational scientists to design experiments that have both a basic science and a translational hypothesis, since then even if the translational component fails, the improved basic science understanding will increase the likelihood that the next translational attempt will be successful.

Which Core Competencies Does a Physician-Scientist Require?

It follows from the foregoing analysis that a physician-scientist performing translational research requires three key skills: (1) the ability to articulate a health need with the precision of a basic science hypothesis; (2) the ability to design a robust and tractable assay (molecular, cellular, organismal, or population-based) to identify potential interventions for further development; and (3) the ability to conceptualize the design of a Phase 3 study to assess the safety and efficacy of the proposed new intervention. All three are required at the start to judge whether to attempt to translate a scientific discovery into improved health in order to avoid mistaken priorities, inappropriate resource commitment, and investigator burnout when unrealistic expectations meet harsh realities.

To articulate a health need with precision requires both an understanding of the state of the art of clinical medicine and deep insight into how to construct a scientific hypothesis. By defining a specific goal, one can judge its potential impact on improving health and then weigh that against the resources that will likely be needed to achieve the goal. In my own career, I built on the knowledge gained from decades of work by others demonstrating a role for platelets in the pathophysiology of acute coronary syndromes and knowledge of the molecular basis of platelet physiology to construct several translational hypotheses: (1) a drug that blocked the platelet $\alpha IIb\beta3$ receptor would improve the therapy of ischemic cardiovascular disease in patients having, or at risk of having, platelet-mediated thrombosis (Coller 1995); (2) monoclonal antibody and DNA-based assessment of platelet $\alpha IIb\beta3$ receptors would facilitate prenatal diagnosis of an inherited disorder of platelet function involving that receptor, Glanzmann thrombasthenia (Seligsohn et al. 1985; French et al. 1998); and (3) bedside monitoring of the effects of antiplatelet drugs on platelet function would improve the efficacy and/or safety of antiplatelet agents (Coller 1998).

Assay design is a vital component of translational research because it allows one to assess the impact of different interventions in search of one or more that can lead to improved diagnosis, therapy, or prevention of disease. Practical considerations such as cost, time required to complete, and complexity are also important, especially if the assay is going to be used to screen large numbers of samples, such as monoclonal antibodies or libraries of organic compounds. The endpoint must be easy to interpret, and the results must be highly reproducible. Most important, it requires the sophisticated integration of both scientific and medical knowledge, since the assay must be medically and biologically meaningful; that is, if the test compound or intervention achieves the desired effect in the assay, it is probable that it will achieve the desired biologic or medical effect when administered to test animals or humans.

In my own research I developed an assay to measure the ability of the platelet $\alpha IIb\beta 3$ receptor to bind fibrinogen by coating small beads with fibrinogen and then determining the ability of platelets to agglutinate the beads (Coller 1980). This permitted me and my colleagues to screen many hundreds of monoclonal antibodies, searching for an antibody that could block the binding of fibrinogen to the $\alpha IIb\beta 3$ receptor on platelets (Coller et al. 1983). One of the antibodies identified (10E5) was used for prenatal diagnosis of inherited disorders of the $\alpha IIb\beta 3$ receptor (Glanzmann thrombasthenia) and another (7E3)(Coller 1985) was later modified in collaboration with scientists at Centocor to become the antiplatelet drug abciximab, which is now used to prevent ischemic complication of angioplasty and stent placement (Coller 1995; Jordan et al. 1996). Subsequent modifications of this same fibrinogen-based assay have been used to screen libraries of organic molecules (Blue et al. 2008) and to develop, in collaboration with the scientists at Accumetrics, a series of point-of-care assays to monitor antiplatelet therapy in clinical settings (Coller 1998; Smith et al. 1999).

To complete a translational project successfully it is necessary to demonstrate the safety and efficacy of the intervention in a rigorous clinical trial. Thus the translational scientist requires knowledge of the steps involved in preclinical development (medicinal chemistry, toxicology, pharmacology, manufacturing), as well as an understanding of how to design and analyze early-phase human studies. In addition, the investigator must have a firm understanding of the bioethical and biostatistical principles that are required to design a pivotal study to establish safety and efficacy. Most important is an understanding of the regulatory process, in particular, selecting a medically meaningful endpoint for the pivotal study that would justify approval for human use. Practical considerations at the interface between academia and the private sector also need to be appreciated, including how the endpoint and number of subjects who need to be studied will translate into the time required to complete the study and the cost of the trial. It also requires an understanding of the goals of the physician-investigators who will recruit the participants and conduct the study, including their desire to advance the therapy of the diseases they treat and their potential concerns about deviating from current standards of medical care. In my own career I was fortunate to have the opportunity to learn from and work with outstanding scientists at Centocor and superb cardiology groups led by Drs. Chip Gold, Eric Topol, Rob Califf, Elliot Antman, and Eugene Braunwald, who provided me with an in-depth understanding of these vital issues (Coller 1995; Coller, Anderson, and Weisman 1995; EPIC Investigators 1994; Antman et al. 1999).

What Should Be the Features and Duration of the Mentored Research Component of Translational Physician-Scientist Training Programs?

Physician-scientists performing translational research need to master three different bodies of knowledge: clinical medicine, basic science, and the design and conduct of human subjects studies to achieve regulatory approval. The first is obtained during medical school, residency, and subspecialty training; the second requires an extended period of rigorous, mentored laboratory research experience; and the third requires a mentored K12 program or its equivalent. It is essential, therefore, that medical students, residents, and fellows considering a career in translational research perceive that there are good opportunities for secure and sustained support throughout this protracted period of training.

For most physician-scientists, the greatest challenge is to obtain rigorous laboratory science skills under the mentorship of an outstanding basic investigator. This experience needs to be long enough for the trainee to learn techniques and develop the intellectual processes required to construct and test hypotheses, and to choose insightfully the appropriate experimental controls. It is extremely advantageous if the environment is encouraging and supportive, helping the trainee ride out the inevitable frustrations that accompany the early phases of a basic science research career. These predictable early failures are particularly ego deflating for accomplished physicians who are used to clinical success and the gratitude of their patients. The trainee must be able to commit at least 75 percent of her or his time to the mentored research project. As a result, it is crucial that clinical activities are organized to complement rather than conflict with the basic science training. A number of practical issues are equally important, including access to nearby affordable housing and day care facilities, and the availability of child care on weekends and holidays for at least brief periods of time so that trainees can attend to crucial time-dependent laboratory tasks such as maintaining cell lines or obtaining timed blood samples. With educational debt compromising the financial security of trainees and adding significant psychological stress, an appropriate salary and loan forgiveness programs are essential elements in attracting and retaining trainees.

The duration of the mentored research experience must be consonant with the reality that the most typical pattern of research productivity for junior physician-scientists consists of a long nucleation process of low productivity followed by a period of exponentially increasing productivity. Thus it is usually very difficult to predict whether a trainee will be successful early in the process. Having adequate support for the last few years may make all the difference in whether a training program succeeds in producing independent scientists.

What, then, is the optimal length of mentored training? This question can be addressed in a number of ways. Since physician-scientists ultimately are expected to compete scientifically against PhD scientists for investigator-initiated grants, it is important to note that most PhD grant applicants have had both four to five years of predoctoral mentored research experience and four to five years of postdoctoral mentored research experience (for a total of eight to ten years). Although MD-PhD students have also had four to five years of predoctoral mentored research experience, MDs who choose a career in translational research after clinical fellowship have often had no more than one year of clinical research experience. Thus a five-year NIH K12, K08, or K23 award is unlikely to provide sufficient experience for an MD to compete successfully. Since a K12 award allows a physician-scientist simultaneously to have a mentored basic science experience and develop skills in translational research methodology, a more appropriate combination might be three years of a K12 award followed by five years of a K08 or K23 award. Currently there is no uniform NIH-wide policy regarding the maximal length of K award support, but most institutes have established a six-year cap. This cap and the variability in NIH institute policies pose problems for mentors trying to advise trainees about entering a K12 program, since participation in the program may prejudice the trainee's subsequent ability to obtain a five-year K08 or K23 grant.

An alternative method for assessing the appropriate length of a mentored research experience is to use existing career development statistics and calculate the number of years between the ages when a typical medical trainee finishes clinical fellowship (~30) and when, on average, an MD investigator is successful in obtaining her or his first NIH R01 grant (~43). Thus, even with eight years of mentored research experience (which would just match in length the mentored experience of PhDs who moved very rapidly through both their predoctoral and postdoctoral experiences), it is likely that the trainee will have to cobble together support for an additional five years before obtaining her or his first R01. At the 2008 K30 and K12 trainee national meeting there was a session on strategies to obtain "bridge funding" to address this reality. Leaving this most vulnerable period to the vagaries of the crazy quilt of "bridge funding" opportunities reduces the likelihood of trainees achieving the status of independent investigators. By analogy, it would be like telling third-year medical students that they have to arrange to get "bridge funding" on their own for their fourth year of medical school.

How Can Physician-Scientists Be Prepared to Understand and Overcome the Cultural Barriers That Separate Clinical Medicine from Basic Science?

Beyond didactic training, academic physician-scientists performing translational research require an in-depth understanding of the cultural differences between basic science and clinical medicine. Appreciation of the cultural differences that exist between academia and industry, and between academia and governmental regulatory agencies, is also important, but I focus on bridging the cultural divide between basic science and clinical medicine because it is the most important for successful translational research. The divide itself originates from differences in orientation and perspective, and is reinforced by differences in training, reward structures, and responses to external pressures. A few examples, exaggerated somewhat to emphasize the contrasts, may help sensitize those on each side of the divide to how those on the opposite side may view them.

The Need for Immediate Action versus Avoiding a Rush to Judgment

Physicians are taught to make decisions rapidly, even if all the data needed are unavailable or ambiguous, whereas basic scientists are taught to reserve judgment until all the evidence is carefully evaluated. Providing medical care to a patient in an emergency requires that the physician accept uncertainty when she or he must act rapidly. In contrast, basic science training emphasizes the importance of eliminating uncertainty, the dangers of coming to conclusions too rapidly, and the need to wait for compelling evidence from multiple experimental sources and multiple approaches before modifying existing paradigms.

Adherence to Standards of Practice versus Encouragement to Challenge Existing Paradigms

Physicians are taught to adhere to accepted methods of diagnosis and therapy, whereas basic scientists are taught to try to supplant current scientific paradigms. Evidence-based medicine, practice guidelines, and the concept of standard of care all reinforce for the physician the importance of following accepted models of practice. Moving away from these norms incurs considerable risk, both from professional colleagues and from patients and their malpractice attorneys should the medical outcome be unfavorable. In contrast, basic scientists are encouraged to challenge current scientific paradigms with bold hypotheses and experiments that provide new mechanistic information that radically transforms the discipline's conceptual model.

Respect for Hierarchy and Expert Authority versus Encouragement to Critique Accepted Wisdom

Physicians are taught to respect the authority of those with more experience and expertise, whereas basic scientists are taught to be skeptical of authority and to challenge it relentlessly. Medical training is organized in variably hierarchical structures, depending on the field, and retains many elements of the apprentice system. Although students and junior trainees are encouraged to ask questions, ultimately they are expected to carry out the plan approved by the senior members of the team. In sharp contrast, basic scientist training emphasizes that all scientific models continuously undergo modification and refinements, and sometimes they are radically overturned by new evidence. Thus, while it is important to study what the current authorities have written and to consider carefully the opinion of one's mentor, it is equally important to constantly probe current models for inconsistencies or inadequacies. Thus the basic scientist is continually looking hard for the weak spots in scientific authority.

Errors as Mortal Threats versus Inevitable Manifestations of the Creative Process

Physicians are taught the importance of developing systems to avoid mistakes, since even the slightest error may have grave consequences for the patient. Each day they face a minefield of potential errors, including incomplete differential diagnoses, drug-drug interactions, disease-disease interactions, and diet-drug interactions, to name just a few. In contrast, basic scientists learn that no matter how carefully they have analyzed the literature and the results of their own previous experiments, many of their hypotheses will not be borne out by their subsequent experiments. In fact many important fundamental discoveries originate as paradoxes. Thus the iterative nature of scientific discovery and the relative ease of repeating most experiments make error less threatening.

The Application of Scientific Knowledge versus the Discovery of Scientific Knowledge

Physicians are commonly taught that they must learn medical science so they can apply the information to improve the health of their patients. By contrast, basic scientists are taught that their job is to create new scientific knowledge.

A Focus on the Unique versus a Focus on the Common

Physicians are trained to look for the unique features in their patient's illness, whereas basic scientists focus on generalizable principles. After their education is complete, physicians readily recognize the common manifestations of disease and begin to devote their attention to identifying unusual features of a patient's illness. The atypical manifestations often reflect interesting genetic or environmental influences, or the presence of coexisting diseases that modify the expression of the illness, and thus they may need to be considered in devising a diagnostic plan and/ or treatment. In some cases the pattern may be so unusual as to suggest an entirely new illness that has never been described. That is why physician-scientists place high value on studying single patients, knowing that many important discoveries that have advanced medical science have come from such careful clinical observations. In contrast, while basic scientists are also on the lookout for paradoxical findings, their orientation is to try to discover general principles through replication, without undue focus on single outlier values that may be the result of many influences, including technical errors. Moreover, the emphasis on the need to replicate results to ensure statistical significance breeds skepticism about "anecdotal" observations.

Uncontrollable versus Controllable Studies

A physician never has the ability to control all variables when analyzing patients. Basic scientists, by contrast, devote enormous effort to devising experiments in which all elements are controlled except the one under study.

Commitment to the Physician's Oath versus Commitment to Search for the Truth

As an integral part of their contract with society, physicians freely profess their commitment to place their patients' interests above their own and to adhere to a high standard of ethical behavior (Miles 2005; Coller, Klotman, and Smith 2002). This oath plays a vital role in defining medical professionalism and consciously or unconsciously constrains the physician-scientist's conception of the boundaries of acceptable scientific inquiry. Although there have been a number of calls to develop an oath for basic scientists (Rotblat 1999; Tsai and Chen 2003; SPUSA 2008), this idea has not met with widespread acceptance because scientists are concerned about imposing boundaries that may limit the intellectual freedom required for scientific inquiry. Basic scientists commonly point to the self-righting nature of science, since truthfulness, reproducibility of findings among different laboratories, and the need for internal consistency are central elements in the scientific process. From the physician-scientist's perspective, while these self-righting mechanisms help to ensure the integrity of scientific data, they do not address the moral dimension, since the next logical experiment from a scientific standpoint may be one that transcends the boundaries of accepted medical ethical behavior (Coller 2006).

Suits and Ties versus Jeans and T-Shirts

Dress is perhaps the most visible manifestation of a culture and commonly clearly differentiates physicians from basic scientists. Physicians are taught that their dress and grooming need to inspire confidence in their patients—or at a minimum not be a distraction. Basic scientists have more freedom to choose clothes and grooming methods on the basis of comfort, affordability, and individual expression—and many take full advantage of the opportunity. Each day the physician-scientist must select clothes reflecting either one or the other culture, knowing that basic scientist attire is not welcome on the wards and that physician attire is likely to produce some raised eyebrows or murmurs in the laboratory.

Perceptions and Frames of Reference

Human perceptions depend on the frame of reference of the perceiver. Thus from the frame of reference of the basic scientist, the physician may seem impatient; too accepting of a hierarchical structure, authority figures, and fragmentary evidence; and conservative in thought, dress, and action. And from the frame of reference of the physician, the basic scientist may seem overly skeptical and reluctant to come to a conclusion; divorced from medical reality; and inappropriately dismissive of the value of single clinical observations. Superimposed on these fundamental differences are economic and lifestyle issues that have the potential to create friction between physician-scientists and basic scientists. Thus basic scientists may envy the higher salaries paid to physicians, and physicians may envy the free tuition and stipends basic scientists receive during their education; their freedom from overnight, weekend, and holiday patient care responsibilities; and their greater control of their working hours.

Having an appreciation of the different frames of reference between basic scientists and clinicians provides insights that can help both trainees and mentors identify the sources of common misunderstandings and potential areas of friction. Thus the leaders of translational research training programs should sensitize both trainees and mentors to the differences in perspective and training so as to develop a climate of mutual respect and trust. A focused emphasis on effective communication, devoid of unnecessary tribal jargon, and explicit articulation of assumptions and specialized knowledge will also help overcome unnecessary barriers and build vital links. These same skills are essential as well for translational research team building, a crucial skill for physician-scientists since no translational project can be brought to fruition by a single investigator.

Do We Need New Career Models and Academic Structures to Facilitate the Development of Physician-Scientists?

The difficulty in recruiting and retaining physician-scientists in translational research careers indicates that we need to rethink our career models and academic structures. For example, two megatrends increasingly affect translational research, namely, the change in the fundamental structure of the American family from one to two careers outside the home, and the need to forge multidisciplinary teams to address complex biologic problems with the goal of improving health. Ignoring the evolution of professional versus family responsibilities has cost the academic enterprise dearly in retaining the best and the brightest. Data described in more detail in other chapters of this book demonstrate that the attrition rate among women entering academic medicine careers is much greater than among men, and the stress of family versus career demands probably accounts for a sizable fraction of male attrition as well.

One possible way to address both of these megatrends simultaneously is for academic medical centers to develop pathways that will allow junior investigators to work as members of cutting-edge, multidisciplinary scientific teams for variably extended periods of time and then encourage them to emerge as fully independent research leaders when their family or other responsibilities allow them to take on all of the administrative and leadership responsibilities that come with being a principal investigator. Such a program would avoid the irrevocable loss of talented young physician-scientists from the translational research pool as a result of their failure to obtain independent funding in an arbitrary time frame. This is particularly important when NIH grants are exceedingly competitive, and the length of federally supported mentored research experiences may not be adequate for even promising physician-scientists to achieve independence. It would also encourage the creation of stable multidisciplinary teams with enthusiastic and highly motivated junior scientists fresh from their mentored training and eager both to make an important scientific contribution and to continue their growth as physician-scientists. The traditional academic system for gaining promotion and tenure is time-limited, so the failure to attain them within a prescribed number of years usually requires the faculty member to switch to a different track or leave the institution altogether. This "up or out" mentality may have had great value in ensuring quality when science was a solitary enterprise and talent could be ascertained rapidly, but now it has become an albatross, forcing arbitrary binary decisions prematurely, with the loss of an enormous pool of human talent. It also drastically diminishes the return on the investment of granting agencies, mentors, and program directors, creating a sense of failure, despair, and frustration.

To succeed, such programs require that academic institutions recognize and reward the junior physician-scientists working in teams for their contributions, including academic advancement and institutional prestige. Especial vigilance is required to make certain that such junior faculty members are not exploited by senior investigators (for example, by usurping authorship), that they are continually encouraged to become independent when the time is ripe, and that they are aided in the process of achieving independence.

Since specialty and subspecialty certification plays such an important role in the career development plans of physician-scientists, it would be valuable to review the certification requirements of the different boards as they affect those considering careers as physician-scientists. In particular, the length of clinical training programs, when coupled with anticipated research experiences, clearly has a negative impact on the desirability and/ or feasibility of a career as a physician-scientist. Creative models that allow physician-scientists to substitute translational research training for traditional subspecialty training, or to integrate the two, are likely to have a profoundly positive effect on the field.

How Can We Develop a New Discipline of Translational Research and a Cultural Identity for the Translational Physician-Scientist?

The CTSA program, referred to at the beginning of this chapter, has helped to make translational research a topic of great interest throughout the United States and much of the world, but there remains confusion as to whether it is simply the name of something that has been done by physician-scientists for decades or whether it truly represents a new discipline. Although it is incontrovertible that many physician-scientists have been conducting translational research for a long time, I am of the opinion that in its modern iteration, translational research meets the criteria for establishing a new cultural identity. I base this on my belief that the skills of translational investigators, regardless of where they stand on the spectrum of bench to bedside (T1) or bedside to curbside (T2), represent both a substantial body of specialized knowledge and a shared series of values. In fact it is particularly important that T1 and T2 investigators better understand each other's disciplines and identify their common goals, since each will benefit, and their translational research efforts will be more likely to succeed. In fact many of the most important successes in translational medicine, such as the development of the statin class of drugs, benefited from data obtained from both T1 and T2 research, with data from T2 studies spurring new hypotheses to be tested by T1 investigators and vice versa.

To facilitate the development of this cultural identity, I have participated in the establishment of a new Society for Clinical and Translational Science (SCTS), with the mission of enhancing the education and science of clinical and translational investigation. The society will co-sponsor with the Association for Clinical Research Training (ACRT) an annual meeting focused on bringing trainees together with junior and senior investigators, as well as other members of the extended family of disciplines that participate in and support translational research. Sessions would focus on trainee education, mentoring, and career development, and would provide a forum for trainees to present their research to colleagues and senior investigators. Other sessions would afford an opportunity for those engaged across the continuum of clinical and translational research to present information about best practices in a variety of disciplines, including new scientific technologies, research nursing, protection of human subjects, bionutrition, trial design and biostatistics, information technology, bio-informatics, research pharmacy, and technology transfer and intellectual property. Other sessions could provide updates on clinical and translational research as viewed by the NIH, the Food and Drug Administration and the pharmaceutical, biotechnology, and contract research organization industries. A plenary session highlighting the best of translational research across the entire spectrum, with introductory comments from leaders in the field to provide historical and scientific perspective, will be an opportunity to learn of the most outstanding advances in the field. The society will also confer awards on trainees, investigators, mentors, government officials, and public advocates for their scientific excellence and/or support of translational research. The society will also sponsor a journal and offer educational information to the public and governmental officials about the field and about the policies and resources required for its sustained growth.

As the society's mission and annual meeting will be crafted to focus on aspects of translational research that are not traditionally the province of existing specialty and subspecialty societies, the discipline of translational research can be viewed as complementing, rather than competing with, the other societies. By meeting and networking together and learning from one another, trainees, investigators, and those involved in the other elements of translational research are most likely to forge a new cultural identity. Ultimately it is the success or failure in creating this cultural identity that is likely to be most important for the future of the field.

5

Women as Physician-Scientists

Reshma Jagsi, MD, DPhil, and Nancy J. Tarbell, MD

One of the most significant changes in the medical profession in recent years has been the dramatic transformation of the demographic composition of its entering members. The gender distribution of the current medical school class now mirrors that of society more generally. Yet women still remain distinctly in the minority on medical school faculties, especially at more senior levels.

One can advance several arguments to support the investigation of gender issues in the physician-scientist community. One argument is deontological in nature. Given that senior positions in academic medicine are among the most highly sought after in our society, gender disparities are of concern simply because fairness dictates that these positions should be open to all. This sort of argument, however, may not be sufficient to convince those who believe that gender disparities are the outcome of freely willed choices on the part of women (ignoring the fact that they play the game on the low side of an uneven playing field).

Therefore it is important also to consider consequentialist arguments. Women constitute an increasingly substantial proportion of the medical workforce, so the continued vitality of the physician-scientist workforce depends critically on the ability of this career to attract the best and brightest minds in medicine, regardless of gender. It also seems reasonable to expect that the increased participation of women in academic medicine would work to the benefit of all in society. Because women have different perspectives and different life experiences from their male colleagues, new ideas and approaches should result from their participation in the academic enterprise. Novel insights are more likely to emerge when individuals of vastly different backgrounds interact. Thus faculty diversity is important for advancing the research, educational, and clinical missions of medical schools. The unique perspective of women may lead not only to greater emphasis on issues of women's health but also to new approaches to disease processes that affect all members of society. Moreover, if young women see the women ahead of them either leaving academics entirely or failing to succeed in advancing to senior positions, they may be discouraged from entering these careers at all, and the potential for their contributions will be lost (Guelich et al. 2002; Andrews 2007). These intergenerational effects must not be underestimated.

In this chapter we discuss the changes in the gender composition of the academic medical workforce in recent years, the challenges and barriers faced by women pursuing physician-scientist careers, the importance of developing a gender-balanced physician-scientist community, and potential interventions to that end.

Demographic Trends

Recent decades have witnessed a tremendous increase in the participation of women in the medical profession. In 2006–7, 49 percent of the applicants to U.S. medical schools and 49 percent of the 17,826 first-year students were women (Association of American Medical Colleges 2008b). As illustrated in figure 5.1, women have also constituted a rapidly increasing proportion of students in combined MD-PhD programs. While the number of men in such programs has remained steady since 1990, the number of female matriculants has increased dramatically, such that nearly all of the growth in the size of these programs has been due to an increase in the number of women (Ley and Rosenberg 2005). Furthermore, women constituted 36 percent of the recipients of mentored research career development awards from the National Institutes of Health (K01, K08, K23 grants) in 1998 but 43 percent of the recipients in 2007 (National Institutes of Health 2008a).

These changes, however, have yet to be mirrored at more senior levels of medical academia, as shown in figure 5.2. In 2007 women constituted 33 percent of all medical faculty (29 percent of basic science faculty and 34 percent of clinical faculty). Yet women constituted only 17 percent of full professors, 11 percent of department chairs, and 12 percent of deans of medical school faculties. Among women holding MD or PhD degrees

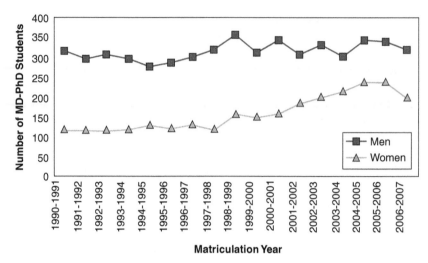

Figure 5.1. MD-PhD students, by gender. Source: AAMC Data Warehouse. Received as a personal communication from Gwen Garrison, PhD, Assistant Vice President, Student and Applicant Studies, March 27, 2008. These data have also been reported by Dr. Timothy Ley. Note: The accrediting body for MD-granting medical schools, the Liaison Committee for Medical Education (LCME), does not require medical school registrars to verify dual-degree students (i.e., MD-PhD). Thus Dr. Garrison notes that she believes the data may significantly underestimate counts through the 1990s by as much as 100 students within the enrollment year. Efforts at the AAMC to improve collection and verification of data on MD-PhD students began in 2002.

in basic science departments, 39 percent were assistant professors, 23 percent associate professors, and 27 percent full professors. Of those in clinical departments, 53 percent were assistant professors, 19 percent associate professors, and 11 percent full professors (Association of American Medical Colleges 2008b). Because many physician-scientists hold MD degrees and not combined MD-PhD degrees, including an important group of so-called "late bloomers" who develop their interest in research careers during or after medical school (Ley and Rosenberg 2005), it is important to consider the dearth of senior female role models for the large pool of potential physician-investigators, as shown in figure 5.3.

Studies of prominent academic journals have shown that women remain in the minority in other highly visible roles in academic medicine as well. Among American MD-authors of original research papers in six major medical journals in 2004, 29 percent of the first authors and 19 percent of the senior authors were female. Women, however, constituted only 11.4 percent of the authors of invited editorials in the *New England Journal of Medicine* and 18.8 percent in *JAMA* in 2004 (Jagsi et al. 2006). Few editors

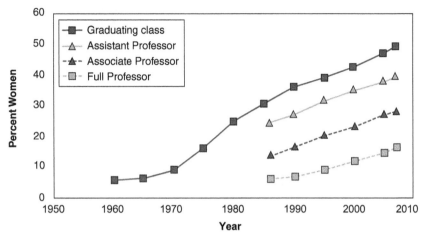

Figure 5.2. Medical school faculty, percentage of women, 1950–2010. Sources: All data from AAMC. Data for medical student graduating class taken from *Women in U.S. Academic Medicine Statistics and Medical School Benchmarking, 2006–2007*, table 1, Medical Students, Selected Years, 1965–2007. Data for faculty in 2007 and 2005 taken from *Women in U.S. Academic Medicine Statistics and Medical School Benchmarking, 2006–2007*, table 3, Distribution of Faculty by Department, Rank, and Gender, 2007; and *Women in U.S. Academic Medicine Statistics and Medical School Benchmarking, 2004–2005*, table 3, Distribution of Faculty by Department, Rank, and Gender, 2005. Data for faculty in 1986, 1990, 1995, and 2000 provided from AAMC Data Book tables and AAMC Faculty Roster system as a personal communication from Le'Etta Robinson, research specialist, Section for Institutional, Faculty, and Student Studies, July 15, 2004. Note: Faculty counts include faculty in basic science and clinical departments. This does not include faculty in departments designated as "Dentistry," "Other Health Professions," "Social Sciences," "Veterinary Sciences," or "All Others."

in chief of major medical journals are female, and women are distinctly in the minority on most journal editorial boards (Jagsi et al. 2008).

Among recipients of competing and noncompeting R01 equivalent (independent investigator) awards from the National Institutes of Health in 2007, 25 percent were women (National Institutes of Health 2008a). A study of grant applications and outcomes at one institution found that observed gender disparities in grant funding were largely explained by gender differences in academic rank (Waisbren et al. 2008). While this study found that, after controlling for academic rank, grant success rates were not significantly different between women and men, it also found that submission rates by women were significantly lower at the lowest faculty rank.

Given these statistics, a debate has developed between those who believe that the low proportion of women at senior ranks is primarily the outcome of a slow pipeline and those who believe that leakage from the

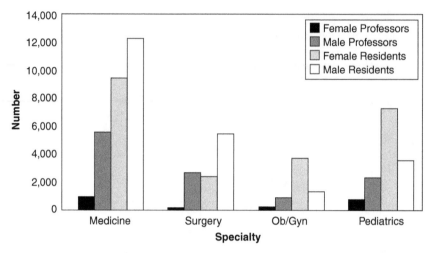

Figure 5.3. The dearth of senior female role models for young physicians in four major specialties. Data are for 2006. Sources: AAMC, *Women in U.S. Academic Medicine Statistics and Medical School Benchmarking, 2005–2006,* table 3, Distribution of Faculty by Department, Rank, and Gender, 2006; and AAMC, *Women in U.S. Academic Medicine Statistics and Medical School Benchmarking, 2006–2007,* table 3, Distribution of Residents by Specialty, 1996, Compared to 2006.

pipeline (be it leakage out of the pipeline altogether or the existence of reservoirs at the lower ranks where women pool and cannot continue to advance) is an additional concern. The "slow pipeline hypothesis" states simply that because women have only recently achieved parity in medical school enrollment, one cannot expect the senior ranks of medical academia to gain immediate parity (Nickerson et al. 1990). Rather one should expect that parity will occur only after women in those medical school classes in which they constitute a substantial proportion of members rise slowly through the ranks from medical student to resident to faculty member. Advocates of this hypothesis note that even after one joins a medical school faculty, there is a particularly long path from instructor to assistant professor and on to associate professor. Finally, the next hurdle is attaining full professorship and the leadership positions associated with that rank. Thus it might take twenty years for a class to advance from medical school matriculation to attainment of full professorship.

Furthermore, individuals remain in the pool of full professors for a number of years after attaining that rank. Therefore it may take additional time for more senior classes, in which the proportion of men is high, to wash out before the proportion of women among full professors (or other senior positions) reaches parity. There are problems with this argument. Today only 17 percent of full professors on medical school faculties are women, even though 24 percent of medical school matriculants in 1975— over thirty years ago—were women. The slow pipeline hypothesis thus seems inadequate to explain the current numbers.

Nonnemaker conducted one of the most thorough and rigorous analyses of these issues to date. She examined rates of advancement of fifteen cohorts of women, graduating from medical school between 1979 and 1993 (Nonnemaker 2000). She found that in the 1980s, the proportion of women entering academic medicine was significantly higher than that of men. This difference, however, was not seen in the cohorts graduating in the 1990s. She also documented that the proportion of women who advanced to the rank of associate professor was significantly lower than expected in all but two of the fifteen cohorts she assessed. Even women who reached the rank of associate professor were less likely to attain the rank of full professor than their male counterparts. Overall, of 519 associate professors attaining the rank of full professor, only 59 were women. The number expected on the basis of their representation in the pool of associate professors was 105—a difference of more than 5 standard deviations. While her findings can be criticized for including all medical school faculty members (including those who are primarily clinically oriented and do not actively seek promotions), they nevertheless provide powerful evidence that the pipeline to seniority is not simply slow but also leaky. In sum, although women's participation in physician-scientist careers is increasing, there is reason to believe that women may face certain gender-related barriers in what appears to be not only a long but also a leaky pipeline to seniority.

Challenges and Barriers

Tesch and colleagues conducted an informative survey study which suggested that differential attrition from academic medicine and differences in productivity are insufficient to explain gender differences in attainment of senior ranks (Tesch et al. 1995). This suggests that women face a number of barriers to advancement that merit further understanding.

Although changes in societal expectations and the law have strengthened women's position in the workforce, some women do continue to face overt discrimination and sexual harassment (Witte, Stratton, and Nora 2006; Stratton et al. 2005; Komaromy et al. 1993). For example, a survey of medical school faculty found that 52 percent of female respondents reported having been sexually harassed by a superior or colleague, compared with 5 percent of male respondents (Carr et al. 2000). Forty-seven percent of the youngest female faculty members surveyed reported experiencing discrimination, as did 70 percent of the oldest faculty. This suggests that discrimination is not yet a thing of the past, despite what one would hope.

Even more common, and potentially more pernicious than overt harassment and discrimination, are subtle, unintentional gender biases. These sorts of biases often originate in deeply ingrained notions of gender roles. Studies have suggested that in our society men may be subconsciously perceived to be natural leaders and innovators, while women may be perceived more often as team members and supporters rather than leaders. This may in turn lead to the disproportionate assignment of plum leadership-building roles, resources, and projects to men. This may then leave women to do far more than their share of patient care, education, and administrative tasks, leaving little time for research and leadership development.

Furthermore, despite data suggesting that the balance between work and family is no more important to women than to men, at least in the younger generation (Dorsey, Jarjoura, and Rutecki 2005; Lambert and Holmboe 2005), department chairs may make subtle subconscious assumptions that women prioritize family over work and may fail to offer certain opportunities to women. Well-intentioned chairs may worry about overburdening female faculty and so unintentionally deprive them of valuable chances to take on responsibilities that are a necessary part of the ascent to leadership.

A report by the National Academy of Sciences details the wealth of social psychological literature demonstrating the pervasive nature of these sorts of gender biases. As it notes, "an impressive body of controlled experimental studies and examination of decision-making processes in real life show that, on the average, people are less likely to hire a woman than a man with identical qualifications, are less likely to ascribe credit to a woman than to a man for identical accomplishments, and when information is scarce, will far more often give the benefit of the doubt to a man than a woman" (National Academy of Sciences, Committee on Maximizing the Potential of Women in Academic Science and Engineering 2006). Indeed such biases may well explain disparities in access to resources, space, salary, and the distribution of awards and other forms of recognition that have been documented in studies such as the landmark study of women faculty in science at the Massachusetts Institute of Technology (Members of the First and Second Committees on Women Faculty in the School of Science 1999).

The effects of subconscious assumptions may be surprisingly powerful. For example, in their striking qualitative study, Yedidia and Bickel recount the experience of a speaker at a medical academic meeting who failed to recognize a woman who stood at a microphone to pose a question until all men (even those not standing at microphones) had made their queries (Yedidia and Bickel 2001). They also report the experience of a woman interviewing for a chair position who was asked by a member of the all-male selection committee: "Are you really sure this is right for your life? Is this really the right thing for you?" One can hardly imagine such a question being posed to a male candidate. Nancy Andrews, the first female dean of the Duke University School of Medicine, noted that many people told her they had assumed she would be unwilling to uproot her family to assume her new position—an assumption that was clearly incorrect. When those recruiting her to the position arranged for the new dean to visit the school her children would attend, the principal immediately reached out to her husband, welcoming him by saying, "You must be the man of the moment" (Andrews 2007). The impact of such assumptions on women who face them, day in and day out, may be quite debilitating.

Gender bias may also be structural and systemic in nature, based in cultural norms and institutional practices that often seem gender-neutral. These ostensibly gender-neutral practices and policies may, however, inadvertently have a negative impact on women. They may create a collision between their biological and professional clocks or magnify the inequities of the traditional gendered division of labor in our society, in which many women continue to bear the greater burden of domestic responsibility. Indeed Carr and colleagues have found that, compared to men and to women without children, women with children face major obstacles (Carr et al. 1998)—and many of these may be rooted in superficially gender-neutral practices.

For example, the common practice of limiting junior investigator grants to individuals within a certain number of years from completion of training may seem to be reasonable, appropriate, and gender-neutral. Such rules, however, inadvertently act to disadvantage women, whose biological clocks may dictate a period of reduced productivity or leave during the training years or immediately thereafter if they wish to have children. By the time these women are able to return to full productivity, many have passed the period of eligibility for training awards.

In recent years a number of the medical specialty licensing boards have articulated more specific policies governing the maximum allowable time away from residency training for childbearing, or have become more active in enforcing already existing policies (Jagsi, Tarbell, and Weinstein

2007). For example, the American Board of Internal Medicine policy re-quires that leave taken in excess of three months during the three years of training for any reason, including vacation and medical leave, must be made up at the end of the training program. Such an extension has finan-cial consequences and may also impact the ability of residents to obtain subsequent jobs or future training positions. Again, these policies may appear to be gender-neutral since they limit the amount of leave allowed to both male and female trainees, but they actually tend to affect female trainees primarily. Although it is true that both men and women may share in parenting responsibilities, only women experience the physically demanding events of childbearing and lactation, which mandate taking a certain amount of leave from work. Parental leave policies that are overly strict or inflexible may therefore have particularly detrimental effects on female physicians.

Some also believe that it is important to consider "sex differences in ca-reer and life goals" in addition to institutional barriers to success (Hamel et al. 2006). It is indeed possible that women have different career pri-orities from men, with women preferring patient care or teaching over re-search, or that women's preferences regarding the balance between work and other activities (such as caring for family) differ from those of men (Buckley et al. 2000; Brown, Swinyard, and Ogle 2003). Yet analyses that emphasize the role of preferences and choice must be careful not to mis-take or define as freely willed the actions of women within the constraints of a gender-structured society. Given the deeply gender-structured na-ture of our society, we believe it is extremely difficult to draw meaningful conclusions based on simple observation of women's choices and prefer-ences. These are in fact necessarily shaped by the constraints women cur-rently face.

Ultimately a complex array of factors contributes to observed sex dif-ferences in academic advancement (Kaplan et al. 1996). Further research regarding the nature and causes of these differences is critical to inform efforts to increase women's representation in the senior levels of academic medicine.

Interventions

Given the disparities observed, the barriers that persist, and the impor-tance of ensuring women's participation in the academic medical enter-prise, the time has come to implement interventions carefully designed to support women in their pursuit of physician-scientist careers. Just as many of the practices and policies that contribute to gender inequity may initially appear to be gender-neutral, strategies to address these issues need not be obviously gender-specific either.

Considerable literature, including studies focusing on academic medicine specifically and studies from other academic disciplines, has demonstrated the value of mentoring for career development (Levinson et al. 1991; Bland and Schmitz 1986; Aisenberg and Harrington 1988; Reich 1986; Roche 1979). These are discussed in detail in chapter 10 by Kenneth Kaushansky and chapter 11 by Alan Schwartz and Margaret Hostetter. Mentoring programs may disproportionately benefit women, even when they are not offered exclusively to women, simply because women may have more to gain from mentoring. Formal mentoring programs may allow women access to opportunities that might otherwise be allocated by an informal "old-boy's network" to which they are not privy. Mentors may also help women understand aspects of the profession and "play games" they never learned in childhood. Mentors may be particularly helpful in showing women how to adapt to the expectations of a profession that has long been male-dominated in its cultural norms (Sirridge 1985).

A number of studies have reported experiences in developing mentoring programs for academic medical faculty (Pololi et al. 2002; Mark et al. 2001; Morzinski et al. 1994) and have sought to identify characteristics of successful mentoring relationships (Jackson et al. 2003; Ramanan et al. 2002). We developed a pilot faculty mentoring program at the Massachusetts General Hospital that vividly demonstrated the potential of such programs to result in benefits for women pursuing careers in academic medicine. In their program evaluations mentees noted the importance of the mentoring relationship in helping them with career planning, balancing work and family, learning about organizational culture, and developing leadership skills. Mentees also noted that the program successfully provided them with a role model and increased visibility (Tracy et al. 2004).

We believe that concerted efforts on the part of academic institutions and professional societies to foster mentoring relationships are necessary. Formal, structured mentoring programs provide a relatively simple and easily feasible way in which to promote the careers of physician-scientists, and particularly the careers of women in academic medicine. The critical importance of mentoring should be rewarded with both institutional recognition and direct financial support of the professional effort involved.

Other concrete interventions may involve the development of grant programs that target women either directly or indirectly, by focusing their support at times of particular need. For example, grants supporting reentry into the academic workforce may be particularly helpful to women who take time away to raise a family but who remain committed to their academic careers (Schubert and Sinha 2004). Thus the design of these awards acts to support women through an otherwise difficult phase for many of them in their careers. Taking a long-term view of physician-scientists' careers and potential contributions, society may thereby avoid the loss of potential that occurs when there is a conflict between women's natural biological clocks and the traditional expectations regarding the timing of faculty productivity over the life cycle.

Another vulnerable time for women physician-scientists is the period immediately after attainment of a faculty position. Some institutions have implemented novel grant programs targeted at junior faculty members. These provide bridge funding explicitly intended to sustain research productivity during the child-rearing years (Emans et al. 2008). A study of early experience with this type of program indicates that the results have been positive. The thirty awardees surveyed reported obtaining a total of $51 million in funding for the direct costs of projects on which they were the principal investigators, dwarfing the $2.1 million institutional cost of the program (Jagsi et al. 2007). Retention was achieved for the majority of awardees, and a large number also achieved promotions. Furthermore, qualitative evidence gathered from participants and their department chairs suggests that the program altered recipients' perceptions of the institution and expectations for a future in academic medicine. The program may even have had a positive impact on the careers of other women at the institution, because awardees reported subsequently advising trainees in their departments on how to manage families and careers. While this experience, as discussed in detail elsewhere, was not implemented as part of a controlled study, we believe that it serves as a model for the type of concrete, targeted interventions that academic institutions should consider.

Other innovative strategies may focus more generally on improving the ability of individuals to balance career with family responsibilities, an issue all physician-scientists face but which may pose particular challenges to female physician-scientists in light of the traditional expectations of our society regarding the gendered division of domestic duties (Okin 1989). The physician-scientist career poses notorious difficulties for those wishing to achieve any sort of work-family balance. This is because long work hours are usually necessary if a physician-scientist is to maintain an active research career and even a modicum of clinical activity. Nevertheless, the Internet and other technological advances have made it possible for many working activities to be completed from home or outside standard working hours. Thus perhaps the current age is fortuitously well suited to the needs of the rising numbers of women entering into physician-scientist careers.

Even where part-time work is not possible, flexible work hours may be extremely beneficial for women seeking to balance work and family (Froom and Bickel 1996). For example, those who wish to leave work in order to see their children before bedtime and to complete their grant writing in the late night hours should not be penalized. This sort of flexibility should be encouraged and supported, with the emphasis on productivity rather than "face time." Important meetings, however, should be conducted during standard working hours, even though many medical professionals have become habituated to expect such meetings to occur in the early mornings and evenings. It is also important for institutions to provide the option of on-site child care in order to minimize the difficulties faced by individuals trying to balance demanding careers with parenthood (Epps and Bernstein 1990). Furthermore, institutions should consider providing financial support that would allow physician-scientists to hire caregivers for their young children when they must travel in their professional capacity.

It is also critical for institutions finally to recognize that—given the differences in biologic needs with regard to childbearing—the course of women's productivity over the life cycle may systematically differ from that of men. Therefore institutions should change the promotion and tenure process to reward contributions without reference to the timing of those contributions. The need for a "tenure clock" should be reevaluated, given its disparate negative impact on female physician-scientists. Systematic interventions to improve awareness of gender issues and to monitor gender disparities are also critical. Department chairs and members of promotions committees should be required to participate in educational sessions regarding the nature of unintentional gender bias. Institutions should provide department chairs and promotion committee members with reports (such as Yedidia and Bickel's analysis and the report of the National Academy of Sciences) in order to ensure that they are aware of the sorts of subconscious biases that may inappropriately influence their deliberations. Annual reviews of department chairs should include explicit discussion of observed gender disparities in resources, salary, and rank among their male and female faculty members (Bickel et al. 2002). Institutions should appoint officers of faculty development with an awareness of these issues and provide resources for programs and speakers to improve the institutional climate with regard to gender issues (Froom and Bickel 1996; De Angelis and Johns 1995).

Reports of interventions that have led to positive outcomes at individual institutions should inspire others to implement similar strategies (Fried et al. 1996). Lessons learned from the National Centers of Excellence in Women's Health, which initiated model programs to promote the advancement of female faculty, should be considered especially carefully (Morahan et al. 2001).

Conclusions

In summary, those concerned with ensuring a high-quality physician-scientist community must be concerned with issues of gender equity. Women constitute a steadily increasing proportion of the overall medical professional workforce, and ensuring that women have equal opportunities to achieve senior leadership positions within academic medicine is critical. A vast body of literature has illuminated the sorts of barriers faced by women pursuing advancement in physician-scientist careers. The time has come for institutions to implement targeted initiatives to help reduce the negative impact of these barriers on women's careers.

All of society loses when a woman in whom many training resources have been invested does not advance. It is the duty of all who are concerned with the mission of academic medicine to ensure that the rising numbers of women entering physician-scientist training paths do indeed have the opportunity to reach their full potential.

6

Generation X and the Millennials in Academic Medicine

DEVELOPING THE NEXT GENERATION
OF PHYSICIAN-SCIENTISTS

Ann J. Brown, MD, MHS

There's a tremendous generation gap between what the current generation of junior faculty want and [what] the current generation of senior faculty perceive as correct.

2003 Duke Faculty Focus Groups, male junior faculty member

The generations queuing up to replace aging baby boomer faculty in academic medicine are different from their predecessors. Whereas boomers are comfortable with total commitment to their careers, Generation X and the millennials will demand a different relationship to work. They will look for environments that support flexible work schedules and policies that support their dual priorities of a stimulating career and time for family and avocations. This raises a question important to those concerned about the future physician-scientist workforce: Will academic health centers (AHCs), with their traditional demand for total devotion to work, be able to continue to attract the most talented individuals from the next generations? With the enormous changes that are affecting AHCs, and by extension the lives of the physician-scientists who populate them, Gen Xers and millennials may well wonder if a career as a physician-scientist, while undeniably compelling, is worth the tradeoffs required. This combination of a changed and changing work environment and the observation that the next generations may not want the same careers as those who went before them suggests an opportunity for AHCs to consider how they will prepare for a future that includes the most talented Gen Xers and millennials.

In this chapter I discuss generational characteristics and explore their impact on the AHC workplace. I then propose professional development strategies for faculty that are tailored to both the changing environment of AHCs and to generational preferences.

Generational Characteristics

According to social science researchers, baby boomers (78 million in the United States) are optimists. Born between 1944 and 1960 into a booming post–World War II economy, they were raised on the message that they would "make the world a better place." In AHCs they occupy senior ranks and leadership positions, where they have brought great ambition to their roles. According to Claire Raines in her book *Connecting Generations* (Raines 2003), boomers have embraced the mission to "make a difference in the world," fueled and exemplified by the civil rights movement, the women's rights movement, and reaction to the war in Vietnam.

Powered by their enormous ambition, boomers "live to work." They tend to define themselves through their jobs and achieve their identity through the work they perform. Their preferred rewards are job-related, and include money, titles, and recognition (Zemke et al. 2000; Brown and Friedman 2007).

Generation Xers (46 million) are described as skeptical. Born between 1960 and 1980, they are our residents and junior faculty. Their boomer parents were so busy at work that Gen Xers became self-reliant. They were the "latchkey kids" who "raised themselves." Having witnessed divorce and downsizing and a roller-coaster economy, they say, "There's more to life than work." High-level public corruption (think Watergate, the Iran-contra affair) taught them to be skeptical of institutions. From these failures of marriage, institutions, and leaders they got the message "Don't count on it," further reinforcing both their self-reliance and their skepticism. In planning their career trajectory, they are more interested in career security than job security. And rather than viewing their career course as progressing along one axis ("climbing a ladder"), they are apt to want to navigate in more than one dimension (perhaps more like rock climbing).

They prize balance between life and work (with the emphasis on the former). With their "work to live" outlook, they are not out to change the world like boomers but instead want a fulfilling life. They are not interested in paying dues to advance (perhaps because they have seen even experienced workers in their parents' generation "downsized"). Instead of years of experience, they want to be evaluated on merit. That does not mean they won't work hard. But they need to be engaged, to see results, and, ideally, to develop portable professional skills through their work. They need "high content and meaning" in work (Kennedy 2003). They expect access to the latest technology, well-developed mentoring programs, and regular and specific feedback (Cornett 2005; Shields and Shields 2003). From a recruiting perspective, they place a high value on a thoughtful orientation.

Gen Xers thus expect family-friendly policies and a controllable lifestyle (Dorsey 2003). They want institutional recognition of their imperative for work-life balance. If they follow the boomer model, they foresee the probability of early burnout. Since they will be in the workforce longer than previous generations, this is not something they can afford to risk. Rewards for them include freedom, time, upgraded resources, opportunities for development, and results for their résumé.

The generation following Gen X, our current medical students and trainees, has been called the millennial generation. Born between about 1980 and 2000 and numbering 77 million, they are described as realistic. They are the children of Gen X and the late-born children of boomers who delayed childbearing or had second marriages. They are adored, and have grown up with involved parents who praised them liberally. They are used to packed schedules and highly structured time, even around play. They are achievement and "brand" oriented, believing that there is a "right" school, program, and career for them and that their task is to amass the necessary credentials to achieve it. They are safety conscious, having grown up in the era of bicycle helmets, seatbelts, and AIDS. They are collaborative, optimistic, inclusive, globally aware, and attuned to multiculturalism. They are a diverse group; as of 2006 nearly 40 percent of millennials aged eighteen to twenty-five were nonwhite (Lopez 2006). This generation has seen terrorism close to home, and for them 9/11 was a defining event. Out of it has come a respect for heroes and a resurgence of patriotism and political interest (Raines 2003; Gale 2007).

They are connected 24/7 via technology. Indeed the Internet has always been an omnipresent feature in their lives, and their technological aptitude has earned them the moniker "digital natives" (with Xers being "digital pioneers" and boomers the "digital immigrants") (Prensky 2005–6). Systems that rely on paper and handwritten documents (such as prescriptions) seem to them hopelessly out of date. They are more identified with technology than any other generation, and for this reason have a lot to offer the workplace. Understanding that their tech skills are needed, they know they are in demand.

They rely on technology to build and stay connected to their communities (e-mail, Facebook, instant messaging, text messaging) and are uncomfortable without this instant access. They have grown up in a culture in which their desires for entertainment, communication, and refreshments can be instantly satisfied online and by ubiquitous sources. Delayed gratification is less familiar and acceptable than it was for previous generations.

More than for other generations, prescription drugs have been part of their life since childhood. They are the first generation to grow up with direct-to-consumer marketing of prescription drugs, which started in 1997. And from a young age they have had personal experience with medications, from antibiotics for ear infections and a myriad of anti-acne treatments to psychotropic drugs. Between 1994 and 2001 prescriptions for antidepressants, stimulants, anxiolytics, mood stabilizers, and antipsychotics more than doubled for adolescents (Thomas et al. 2006).

At work, millennials are looking for good leaders (perhaps to re-create their highly managed childhoods). They are looking for workplaces that provide excellent orientation and strong mentoring (being similar in this way to Gen Xers). They want to be challenged, to enjoy their work and their colleagues, and to be treated with respect from day one (Raines 2003). Being technologically savvy, they are used to finding information nearly instantly, and to being able to work anywhere, anytime. Having been raised with e-mail and text messages, they are used to communicating in "bullet points not paragraphs" (Gale 2007). This often translates into casual or informal—and grammatically incorrect—written communication, which can be a source of tension, as it may be perceived by others as disrespectful. They may undervalue face-to-face communication (Gale 2007) and be impatient with tasks requiring more extensive discussion. While they enjoy working with friends, they tend to build fewer ties in the workplace. Loyalty is to self, social networks, and career, not institution.

Like Gen Xers, they value flexibility and look for work environments that recognize their multifaceted interests, including family, community service, and avocations. They expect policies that allow generous leaves and vacation, and a workplace that stays current with the latest technology. They may respond to nonmonetary rewards such as time off, upgraded technology, or professional development opportunities. Being used to liberal praise for any effort, they may need clear explanations about the amount of work required to achieve a particular outcome. Taking time to point out what a task will teach them, and how the skills acquired will benefit them, may be especially useful in motivating this generation.

Their considerable energy can also be harnessed through ample, frequent, and personalized feedback. This, when linked to clear explanations of the intended outcome of their work (both for themselves and for the employer), provides an important framework for managing this generation. Thus senior faculty and administrators need to have skills in setting clear objectives, explaining the big picture, taking the time to give regular and prompt feedback, and ensuring that millennials feel valued and successful.

Generations in Academic Medicine

"It is naïve," writes one researcher, "to assume that the traditional medical career structure, in which a strong sense of vocation drives an individual to selflessly work long hours in substandard conditions, will re-emerge as the dominant model or is a viable solution to current medical workforce problems" (Skinner 2006).

How do the different generational traits, culled from research on a wide cross-section of the U.S. workforce and not specifically targeting physician-scientists, apply to academic health centers? In recent years a number of authors have suggested that indeed, even though physicians and faculty are a highly selected group with strong motivation for professional work, generational differences are operating.

Boomers

For boomer physicians, their commitment to medicine is total. They see themselves as MDs first and have thrived in an environment that demands their total effort. Traditional physician-scientist careers seem perfectly tailored to this preference. Boomers "define professionalism predominantly in terms of hours worked and 'complete' dedication to the job. Baby boomers, creating a value system based on their own life ethic, have confused work ethic with professionalism. Still in charge of the academic medical system, baby boomer physicians have continued to enforce a workplace that demands long hours, total dedication to work, rigid approaches to patient care, and disdain for anyone who does not accept their 'rules of life'"(Smith 2005).

But for boomers, the profound dedication to work may be reaping fewer rewards than in the past as profound changes alter the landscape of faculty life in AHCs. Focus groups of senior faculty at the author's institution describe escalating time pressures, a growing emphasis on budget management, and the need to comply with increasingly complex regulations (Bickel and Brown 2005). Declining clinical reimbursement means that faculty must perform more clinical services to generate the same revenue. All of these changes threaten precious time for research and for activities that rely on flexible time such as teaching, mentoring, and informal networking.

"I think it is much worse now for all of us," said a senior male faculty member in a 2003 focus group. "We just don't have the time we used to have. Nobody has the time. I used to have a half to a third of my academic day where I could go and do something with somebody. And now, the pressure to basically produce is so extensive and so horrible in a sense, that you just don't have time to basically talk to people at the end of the day.... [W]e're all making about the same amount of money, but we're all 30 to 40 forty percent busier." He added: "Previously we had lower salaries and more free time. Now junior faculty are pushed so hard to generate salary that there is no free time" (Bickel and Brown 2005).

Generation X

Whereas boomers are apt to view being a physician as their identity, Gen Xers consider this one of the many things that define them (Kennedy 2003). Gen X has experienced firsthand the cost to personal health and family integrity of boomers' overarching dedication to work. Gen X physicians, like their nonmedical colleagues, value time for avocations and family and want job flexibility, autonomy, and a solid income (Skinner 2006).

These priorities were confirmed in a survey of recent graduates of doctoral programs (not necessarily in medicine) who were anticipating academic careers. As they prepared to launch their careers as faculty, among their top five priorities were time for family and personal obligations, and a flexible work schedule (Trower 2007). This preference is also noted in surveys of younger physicians. In a 2006 survey conducted by the AAMC, 71 percent of physicians under age fifty cited time for family and personal pursuits as a very important characteristic of a desirable practice (Kirch and Salsberg 2007). One tangible example of these values in the medical workforce is a growth of hospitalists. This specialty, in which physicians limit their practice to inpatient care, has been called the fastest-growing specialty in history (Kralovec et al. 2006). For the younger generations, the hospitalist combination of meaningful work, regular work hours, and good compensation is highly attractive.

This preference for controllable hours grates on some boomers. One example of this is the July 2003 implementation of the eighty-hour workweek limit for residents and fellows, which has stirred up considerable debate about the work ethic and professionalism in medicine. Senior faculty have questioned whether the next generation of physicians, raised on "shift work," will have the commitment to meet the demands of the profession.

In this context it is worth noting that one reason why Gen Xers may need controllable hours is that their lives at home are different from those of their boomer mentors. For many senior faculty role models, successful careers were built on the premise of their unlimited availability for work, supported by a full-time unpaid household manager (usually a wife). Now two-career couples are common, particularly for women physician-scientists. Both partners struggle, with minimal assistance from their institutions, to balance the competing demands of work and life outside of work. Choosing a job with controllable hours is one way to mitigate that struggle.

Despite the sharp distinctions in how boomers and Gen Xers perceive and are perceived, they may actually put in the same hours. In a study of boomer and Gen X faculty in a Canadian medical school, both generations felt that the younger faculty were seen as less committed to their careers and as having an anemic work ethic. When asked to report their hours spent at work and at home, however, both groups reported working identical hours per week, suggesting that perception and reality may be different (Jovic et al. 2006).

Millennial Generation

While the millennial generation is still making its way through medical training programs and has not yet entered the faculty ranks, the traits of its members suggest that they may be well suited to careers as physician-scientists. Their lifelong achievement orientation may be an excellent preparation for the challenging training process and for the achievement-oriented career that follows. And the professional objectives of such a career will appeal to their aspiration to do work that is meaningful (Howe and Strauss 2007). But they are likely to want to see some aspects of the academic work environment adapted to their preferences.

What is known about millennial medical students and their career preferences? They will opt for careers with a controllable lifestyle—a preference not countermanded by their achievement orientation (Dorsey et al. 2003). Some authors have commented that these seemingly opposing desires for flexibility and high achievement make millennials look like they "want it all" (Nelson 2007). Indeed their skills at multitasking, savvy use of technology, and fluid work-life boundaries may give them confidence that they can actively pursue multiple agendas simultaneously and seamlessly. Given these traits, we are unlikely to see a return of the boomer style workforce, where occupation and identity were so deeply enmeshed.

In imagining the fit between academic work and millennial skills, it is clear that this cohort has traits that are in demand in the world of academic research. Described as "sociable" and "connected" and liking to work toward specific goals and in collegial groups, millennials may bring a much-needed ability to work effectively in collaborative units. As scientific inquiry evolves quickly toward "big science," with large-scale studies (Ginsburg et al. 2008), and multidisciplinary and multi-institutional collaborations, scientific careers will demand more work in large teams. The social networking skills that millennials bring with them to the workplace will be useful in responding to the powerful trends in scientific inquiry.

To extrapolate again from millennial characteristics to the academic workplace, it is likely that millennials will do their best work in environments that engage active management practices. Raised with involved parents who orchestrated a full schedule of achievement-oriented activities, and praised them liberally, millennial physician-scientists may look for parallel leadership styles at work. They will respond well to structured environments, clear lines of authority, and clear goals (Howe and Strauss 2007). To put this another way, a research lab or department that works well for self-directed and self-reliant Gen Xers may work less well for millennials.

There will likely be specific challenges around communication. The millennial preference for electronic messaging may frustrate older co-workers more accustomed to the fuller range of communication tools available in face-to-face discussions, such as facial expression, tone of voice, and cadence. Millennials will question the traditional emphasis in academic environments on "face time," and push for more emphasis on evaluations based on competence and not time in training or time spent at work. Thus, to make the most effective use of millennial talent, senior faculty and other AHC leaders will need to hone management skills that can be tailored to different styles and values. Since academic leaders are not commonly trained in management skills, management training may be an important innovation to help bridge generational gaps.

The inherent reliance of AHCs on competition to achieve excellence may also be a point of tension with millennials. The celebrated "sink or swim" environment, with an "up or out" tenure system, may seem peculiar (and thus uninviting) to millennials. Having been raised with electronic games, in which a key to success is knowing the rules, they may find it irksome to navigate a career environment in which rules are less clearly codified. Having grown up in an environment of praise, where even small achievements are celebrated, and where everyone can be successful, millennials may have little tolerance for the idea that some are more talented than others. They have been raised to expect success, and may be inexperienced at dealing with disappointments such as not matching at a first-choice residency, or having a grant rejected, or any other indication that their best may not be good enough. Their upbringing may make it tough for them to find a highly competitive and purposefully ambiguous AHC environment appealing.

Competing Successfully for the Next Generations

Academic research careers, no matter how compelling, may look uninviting to the younger generations. They may be seen as offering too little opportunity for work-life balance, too much dependence on delayed gratification, too much frustration if grants are not funded and papers not accepted, and too much reliance on career strategies that worked better in a different era. What changes will prepare AHCs to recruit and retain the most talented men and women of Generation X and the millennial generation? An overarching theme that will appeal to their generational characteristics is investment in junior faculty that is visible and systematic (but personalized), with emphasis on career management skills. Three top items should be flexible work options supported by accommodating policies, creative mentoring programs, and management training for leaders.

Flexible Work Options

Academic careers inherently have a certain amount of flexibility, but this valuable quality could be enhanced and made more systematically accessible. For more uniform—and equitable—availability, and in order to leverage meaningful support for such issues as child care and tenure clock extensions, institutional engagement and support is essential. Table 6.1 lists examples of the types of policies and practices that many younger faculty will look for. Whether or not they are highly used policies, at minimum they signal that the institution recognizes the multigenerational needs of their faculty workforce and supports them.

Policy implementation is, however, only the first step. It must be accompanied by a cultural change that smoothes the way for these policies to be used by both men and women, and without the stigma of appearing less serious about one's career. Frequent communication from leadership about the availability of policies, and statements of philosophical support for their use, are important catalysts for this cultural change.

Building flexibility will require other cultural changes as well. It will demand a high degree of faculty-faculty and faculty-staff cooperation—perhaps more than is typical for an environment that primarily rewards

Table 6.1. Policies and strategies to support work-life balance

Policy	Features
Promotion policies	• Defined tracks for promotion that recognize different types of work and scholarship • Recognition of interdisciplinary team science • Availability of "undeclared" status for new faculty to allow time to decide on career path
Flexible and part-time work arrangements	• Full-time employment status with modified work duties and possibly reduced work hours • Maintenance of benefits • Ability to remain on the tenure clock • Tenure clock relief • Temporarily modified duties during pregnancy if needed • Job-sharing options • Sabbatical leave
Tenure clock relief	• Covering a spectrum of life events, including childbirth; adoption; caring for spouse, domestic partner, parent, child, or other family member; personal illness; or medical disability • Pursuing advanced degree or certificate • Administrative load
Leave policies	• Paid and unpaid leave options • Parallel with tenure clock relief polices, covering a spectrum of life events, including childbirth; adoption; caring for spouse, domestic partner, parent, child, or other family member; personal illness; or medical disability • Pregnancy disability • Pursuing advanced degree or certificate
Technology that supports flexibility around learning, meeting, and working	• Teleconferencing • Podcasts/Webcasts • Data accessibility from remote locations for patient care and research • Social networking software
Dependent care assistance	• On-site care, sick-child care, institutional collaboration with local child care facilities, financial assistance • Early childhood education programs • Lactation rooms • Travel funds for parents who must bring children to research conferences (e.g., for breastfeeding) or hire help while away • Elder care assistance • Adoption benefits
Employee assistance programs	• Short-term psychological counseling • Physical fitness resources • Financial counseling resources
Academic reentry programs	• Assistance for reentering workforce after absence (e.g., for child rearing)
Concierge services	• Assistance with personal services (errands, shopping, travel, home or car maintenance, etc.)
Dual career accommodation	• Assistance with job search for partner • Relocation assistance

individual achievement. Flexible work arrangements, including any shift work or job-sharing measures, will require effective cross-coverage strategies, which in turn will require tools for effective communication, and a spirit of collegiality (Goldstein 2008). Teaching communication and teamwork skills, both in the laboratory and in clinical care, will support this cultural change and is inherent in the faculty development strategies discussed next.

Another generational benefit of these policies is worth mentioning here. Policies tailored to the needs of younger faculty can help develop institutional loyalty. While boomers can build strong ties to institutions out of their love of work, Gen Xers and millennials, cautious about trusting organizations, may need additional incentives, such as those provided through the policies outlined in table 6.1. To extend this idea further, programs that help link people to institutional treasures such as gardens, museums, architectural gems, exercise facilities, and sports teams may create a sense of pride and loyalty. By encouraging faculty to enjoy these assets, an institution can send a message designed to resonate well with younger faculty (particularly millennials) that "we want you here."

Faculty Development Programs

With increasingly constricted time for unfunded activities such as mentoring, and the complicated process of learning to function at full capacity in a new environment, a structured faculty development program can be an excellent way to support junior faculty. But in order to be effective, programs must be designed to go beyond a simple recommitment to traditional mentoring and must incorporate strategies that appeal to generational sensibilities.

For instance, junior faculty need tools to help them quickly demystify academic careers and institutional processes. This requirement flies in the face of the more confidential and "need to know" approach that is familiar to older generations. Senior faculty are as a rule more accustomed to decisions being made "behind closed doors," in ways that protect privacy and ensure candor (Trower 2007). Programs that explain the ground rules are an investment in faculty, and their existence is tangible evidence that the institution values its junior faculty. This is a feature that appeals particularly strongly to millennials, who need to know that they are valued.

Explaining the rules also appeals to the millennials' preference for clear instructions and helps address their low tolerance for ambiguity. They may feel more equipped to respond with their best when they have a clear understanding of the task being asked of them, with all of its steps and goals. They may also appreciate efforts to clarify the link between their current work and a future that holds the success they are looking for. Thoughtful and personalized explanations may aid them in persevering through the inevitable failures that occur in building academic careers. Letting them know that manuscript rejections, for instance, are expected occurrences, and giving guidance on how to respond, may be critically important tasks in mentoring millennial fellows and junior faculty. For senior faculty providing this mentorship, it is worth recalling that many of the processes of academic medicine are not obvious to novices. Taking the time to explain even basic procedures may be enormously helpful.

Skill development seminars are a key element of faculty development programs. Well-conceived seminars can shorten the ramp-up time for acquiring needed skills such as grant writing, public speaking, and conflict management (Aschwanden 2008; Wingard et al. 2004). And using interactive learning (rather than the "sage on stage" strategy) can effectively build a sense of community and appeal to the millennial preference for working in collegial groups (Howe and Strauss 2007). These programs may also appeal to younger generations' orientation toward "results" and their enthusiasm for augmenting their career security by building their portfolio of portable skills.

While traditional one-on-one mentoring will always be important (Keyser et al. 2008), alternative ways of learning organizational culture and career conventions will be vital for generations uneasy with institutions and hierarchy. For instance, peer mentoring, in which groups of peers work together to address professional development challenges (Moss et al. 2008), can serve as a way to build networks for social support and for information sharing. Such networks could also address the challenge of connecting the growing numbers of nonmajority scientists (women, ethnic and racial minorities, foreign scientists, lesbian/gay/bisexual/transgendered individuals) to an institution full of colleagues and leaders who do not look like them.

Group mentoring, in which one or two senior faculty members facilitate a cadre of junior faculty that meets as a group, may also be appealing (Pololi et al. 2002). Managed appropriately (which might require training of the senior facilitators), the groups can engage junior and senior faculty in ways that dilute the intensity of the chain of command. By reducing the emphasis on any one individual, groups can facilitate candid cross-generational communication and build understanding. This "one-to-many" model offers the additional potential advantage of reducing the time burden on any single senior faculty member.

The traditional dyadic senior-junior mentoring relationship can also be revitalized in potentially simple ways. For instance, mentors who approach their mentee more like an encouraging parent or coach and less like an intimidating authority figure may find millennials more receptive. Mentors can defuse tension by acknowledging up front that their mentee may need to forge a different pathway to success than they did. Mentors should not assume or expect deep similarities with their mentee. This may require surrendering the historically invigorating idea that by mentoring, a mentor will establish someone who will "follow in his footsteps." Instead the reward will come from reaching across differences to help someone harness his or her own motivation and maneuver his or her unique life circumstances to achieve success.

Programs like those highlighted in boxes 6.1 and 6.2 can address many organizational needs, including the need for faculty to get to the point of success quickly, however defined by the institution. At the same time, designed with generational sensibilities in mind, these programs can also be tremendously appealing to Gen Xers and millennials, and thus be useful tools for recruitment, retention, and performance management.

Management Training for Leaders

The process used to choose academic leadership has been described as "accidental" (Collins-Nakai 2006). Academic leaders are traditionally

---

Text Box 6.1

According to Tom Cech, president of the Howard Hughes Medical Institute (HHMI), "assistant professors are hired based on their scientific research accomplishments, but their success as faculty members is very much related to their ability to manage a small business" (Aschwanden 2008).

To address this gap in training and to help investigators "hit the ground running," HHMI partnered with the Burroughs Wellcome Fund to develop a lab management curriculum. This curriculum focused on skills such as making hiring decisions, mentoring, providing performance evaluations, giving appropriate feedback, managing conflict, budgeting, obtaining research funds, writing grants, and time management. It has been adopted at several institutions and been well received. Trainees and junior faculty appreciate the opportunity to develop career skills that reduce the "trial and error," "sink or swim" approach to acculturation.

Text Box 6.2

The University of California, San Diego, School of Medicine developed a seven-month curriculum for junior faculty members, each selected through a competitive process (Wingard et al. 2004). The curriculum included a series of workshops, career planning sessions, individual academic performance counseling sessions, formal senior-junior mentoring relationships, and network building. Each class spent much of an academic year together and developed collegial relationships. Compared with pre-program ratings, graduates were 52 percent more confident in their abilities in professional development, 20 percent more confident in their research capabilities, 33 percent more confident in their education skills, and 76 percent more sure of their administrative responsibilities. In addition to being perceived by participants as increasing their self-efficacy, the return on investment was a substantial 49 percent, indicating that the institutional investment in the program was financially sound.

chosen for their scientific achievements, not necessarily their management skills. Any skill they have in this realm is, in this construct, "accidental." But with increasing organizational complexity and intensifying demand for financial and interpersonal expertise, management skills are more important for leaders than ever before (Korschun et al. 2007; Souba 2004).

From a generational perspective, effective leadership resonates as a significant distinguishing feature in AHCs. Having grown up with "helicopter parents," millennials in particular are comfortable with someone being in charge (as long as that "parental figure" is admiring, encouraging, and concerned for their success rather than authoritarian or judgmental). Millennials and Gen Xers are likely to look for leaders who reach out to them to understand their perspectives and work styles. They will appreciate leaders who recognize generational penchants, such as the preference for electronic communication, less emphasis on "face time," transparency of processes, organizational support for collaboration, and flexibility around work hours. They will particularly need leaders who are skillful at communicating about career progress, help them see a successful future, and create opportunities to provide constructive and detailed feedback. They will value leaders who have the skills to manage people effectively, particularly those who prefer a nontraditional approach to their careers.

Interpersonal skills may be especially important for leading Gen Xers and millennials. Because these groups are characteristically wary of institutions, leaders must work to build trust, a task that requires skillful communication. Gen Xers and millennials appreciate leaders who convey an interest in understanding them, and who express a willingness to work with the value systems they bring. Gen Xers and millennials expect ethnic, racial, and gender diversity, and they expect leaders to be conversant with how bias, including unintentional bias, operates in the workplace.

They also look for clear statements about the value of the variety of faculty career paths needed to operate a modern AHC. In addition to the traditional emphasis on research, younger generations are looking for institutional rewards for activities such as teaching, mentoring, and institutional service (Trower 2007). Such rewards could include, in addition to financial compensation when available, creation (or expansion) of teaching and mentoring awards. These awards should acknowledge work in all arenas (research, clinical, teaching, and administrative) that are vital to the institution. They should also be linked with processes that help build a community of scholars in that arena (such as a mentoring academy). Good leaders will be able to communicate clearly about the value of these activities.

Skillful leadership need not be "accidental," nor should AHCs rely on less than excellent leadership to guide faculty through the tempest of building academic careers. To this end, investment in leadership training for faculty, with a strong emphasis on communication skills and understanding and respecting generational differences, is a key element for any strategy to recruit and retain the next generations of academic physicians.

Conclusion

In this chapter I have described factors affecting faculty and trainees in AHCs today, viewed through the lens of generations. There are clearly developmental factors other than generational group that influence the character of the emerging physician-scientist workforce. The focus in this chapter on generation is not meant to discount the influence of gender, race, ethnicity, sexual orientation, region or country of upbringing, socioeconomic class, or any of a number of other forces that affect choices and behavior. In addition, it is worth mentioning that some authors question the premise of categorizing groups based on birth year (Giancola 2006), pointing to the dearth of peer-reviewed publications on this topic. Nonetheless, the generational construct may provide a useful (if incomplete) framework for understanding changes affecting the AHC work environment.

By considering how a generation—a group that experiences similar large-scale historical events as its members mature into adulthood—might approach their careers, we may gain useful ways of interpreting, responding to, and predicting their behavior.

To summarize, both societal norms and the academic workplace are changing, and doing so rapidly. Financial pressures are more front and center than in the past, and faculty are increasingly obligated to comply with institutional, government, and payer demands. In this context there is the perception of diminished discretionary time and dollars. Yet coming generations are looking to "have it all," including competitive salaries, flexible work options, and controllable lifestyles. In this scenario the imperative for institutional belt-tightening stands in apparent conflict with the generational demand for flexibility, creating a further economic challenge for institutions.

The opportunity for activities that rely on flexible time, such as mentoring, has contracted in this environment, leaving new faculty with fewer resources to navigate the choppy waters. This suggests that institutions must champion deliberate efforts to provide faculty support in a systematic way. These efforts should include the provision of policies that support work-life balance, faculty development programs that teach skills and use creative mentoring strategies, and management training for leaders. Such initiatives would be geared to helping faculty navigate their institution and build successful and rewarding careers. By being highly accessible to all faculty, particularly the growing number of women and minorities in the next generations, such efforts will help AHCs engage the full pool of available talent. Engagement of the next generations, informed by an awareness of group characteristics that may arise from their unique socialization, will be critical to the future success of the physician-scientist workforce.

7

Engaging Undergraduate Students in Research

SUSTAINING OUR NATION'S PIPELINE OF FUTURE BIOMEDICAL INVESTIGATORS

Stephen G. Emerson, MD, PhD, Philip Meneely, PhD, and Jennifer Punt, VMD, PhD

As the twenty-first century opens, the potential for biomedical research to yield meaningful discoveries that enhance human health and mitigate disease is clearly greater than ever before. Targeted therapeutics, tissue engineering, genotype-selective diagnostics, and many other new fields beckon. Making the most of these exciting opportunities will require physician-scientists who are as excited by these possibilities as they are trained to contribute to the development of these fields. So while it is clearly important to ask, "How do we keep interested physician-scientists in the field?" it is equally and perhaps more useful to ask, "How do we best entice, educate, and train undergraduates to enter the physician-scientist pathway in the first place?"

In this chapter we offer one perspective on undergraduate training for careers in biomedical research, that is, creating the human capital entering the field. This perspective is based on our experiences studying and teaching at Haverford College, an early, continuing, and disproportionate source of successful MD-PhD and research-focused MD scientists. From each graduating class of three hundred students, approximately three or four per year (5 percent of all science majors, 1 percent of all Haverford graduates) enter combined degree programs. Another 5 percent of graduates enroll in biomedical PhD programs without enrolling in medical school, and an additional 5 percent enter medical school alone, but with a strong interest in research careers. These experiences, combined with our careers spanning graduate and postgraduate research training at the National Institutes of Health (NIH), national research institutes, and research-intensive professional schools, have taught us several key lessons about critical rate-limiting steps in the progression to a career as a physician-scientist.

Undergraduate Science Curricula Should Be about Laboratory Discovery

We believe that to successfully recruit talented students into a biomedical research career, we must inspire them and show them how intellectually challenging and exciting is the actual practice of research. As our biology curriculum has continued to evolve along with the progress of science itself, our belief has been that experimental thinking and laboratory investigation are primary; everything else is built to support that experience.

Our guiding principle at Haverford is that—from the outset of their academic experience—all students are treated as prospective investigators. As they proceed through the curriculum, they are led progressively to gain independence at the bench. This experience culminates with year-long research theses under the aegis of research-active faculty mentors. This training is not primarily focused on the technical skills associated with laboratory research, although that is a necessary component. Instead the research training focuses on the intellectual aspects of research—posing experimental questions, assembling and interpreting data, offering oral and written presentations, and planning the next experiment. Therefore the process of thinking about research begins not in the senior year but during the students' first introductory coursework in cell and molecular biology. Laboratory experiments are hypothesis-based, heavily interpreted, and often open-ended.

At Haverford College students experience their first biology course as sophomores. Because the curriculum is based in cell and molecular biology, students are required to take undergraduate chemistry either before or concurrently with the biology courses. As soon as they begin these courses, students are asked to see themselves—and to think as—individuals who are collecting and analyzing experimental data. They are challenged to ask: "What was the experiment that supported those claims, how was it performed, and what were its critiques and limitations? What else could have been done to build a better, richer argument?"

The junior year builds on this experimental approach by centering on stand-alone lab courses in the chemistry and biology departments known affectionately as "Superlab." This series of four quarters features modern experimental approaches and techniques (e.g., molecular cloning,

RNAi, expression array profiling, NMR, atomic force microscopy, flow cytometry) that explore areas currently under investigation in the literature. With strong guidance by faculty with expertise in the field, students design, execute, interpret, and often publicly present their own experiments. From the perspective of bench investigators, they read and interrogate relevant primary literature and so already begin to see their own work as part of a larger, exciting scientific community.

Supporting this core laboratory experience are advanced topics courses in cellular and molecular biology (e.g., genetics, biochemistry, cell signaling, immunology, developmental biology molecular neurobiology, microbiology) that begin to expose students to primary data in historical and current literature while extending the intellectual scope and mastery of the student. Coursework culminates in a series of senior-level seminars in which students publicly critique the literature in a field of current importance (e.g., stem cell biology, apoptosis, aging, nanotechnology) in a class that can best be described as a mentored journal club.

The summer between junior and senior years marks the beginning of many students' senior research thesis projects. This work, performed by every senior major, occupies the core of the senior year experience and is performed with faculty members in their laboratories. Students commit between ten and twenty hours per week in the lab, receiving credit for this experience. Students work closely with their mentors on projects that are related to the faculty member's own funded work. The process, however, explicitly encourages students to develop original perspectives, approaches, and questions—resulting in a thesis that is informed by faculty experience but distinctly "owned" by the student. It is routine for students basically to inhabit their mentor's laboratory, and not uncommon to see lights on in the lab late into the night. Through this process, all students produce sufficient experimental work to create a coherent poster for presentation at regional, national, or international meetings. Students generally attend these meetings and present their own posters. Most of their work is directly incorporated into peer-reviewed publications from the faculty's laboratories.

We should add that a vital part of this process is mentoring. Faculty function as enthusiastic, challenging, but optimistic cheerleaders for their students. Simultaneously, students see their faculty engaging in the full spectrum of professional activities: presenting at meetings; writing and reviewing manuscripts; writing and receiving grants from the NIH, NSF, HHMI, and other institutions; troubleshooting new techniques. Not surprisingly, one of the advantages for students at Haverford and similar small colleges is that they are in direct intellectual proximity with their faculty mentors. Without graduate students and only rarely with post-docs, undergraduates are at the front lines themselves.

By the time students graduate, they have seen themselves begin to think and successfully function as bench scientists. Because they pursue this path in the company of colleagues, they see research as a normal, challenging, but also—and this is critical—realistically attainable life activity. A research career appears as one that is compatible with everything else in their lives, from a broad range of academics, to intercollegiate athletics, to drama and art, to friendships and family. Rather than wondering, "What hoops must I jump through before I can become a happy, successful, fulfilled scientist?" they are more likely to think, "I really enjoy being a scientist already." It is important to note that much of the success of this program lies in expos-ing all majors to a research-focused curriculum. Some students who had not considered research find themselves enjoying the ownership of an idea and project; some who may not have thrived in the classroom find themselves in their element in the laboratory. Nevertheless, and perhaps most important, all majors, regardless of their career aspirations, become part of a natural community of scholars.

Interdisciplinary Scientific Coursework Should Prepare Students to Become Analytic Interdisciplinarians

How do we train and inspire young students to thrive in an environment that is changing at a rapid pace and becoming increasingly interdisci-plinary and technologically driven? Clearly tomorrow's biomedical in-vestigators will need to be comfortable working with chemists, computer scientists, and engineers, among other professionals. Even more impor-tant, they will need to know both when to work with scientists in such disciplines and how to lead and guide effective collaborations. We believe that such training and habits should begin early, and that this makes for the most vibrant and productive experience for students and faculty alike.

Over forty years ago the Haverford biology faculty realized that their students needed to understand organic and physical chemistry in order to approach cell and molecular biology with the proper sophistication. As the needs of the active researcher have changed with each new discov-ery, this belief in interdisciplinarity has evolved over the years. Physical and organic chemistry and physics continue to underlie and support bio-logical research. Perhaps the most interesting interdisciplinary develop-ment in recent years, however, has been the reintroduction of mathematics and computer science into the foundations of research biology. In a sense, biology has come full circle as computational approaches have reasserted the importance of phylogeny and evolutionary biology, albeit through "in silico" eyes. Sequence homology comparisons, expression array profiling with its layers of analytical approaches, and mathematical modeling of interacting signal transduction pathways are all essential components in the new conversations about emergent behavior of complex systems—that is, systems biology. These areas require some familiarity with approaches in statistics and probability, and arguably with linear algebra and Fourier transforms. In addition, the application of (slightly) more complex mathematics to traditional physical chemistry formulae has led to broad insights from the biology of complex tissues to biological sustainability. Of course we do not believe that all of our biology students, nor all future physician-scientists, need to be mathematicians or computer scientists. Rather we believe that many of the underlying computational principles for contemporary biology are grounded in mathematics that is accessible to nearly all students, and not only to those who are the most mathematically inclined.

We have also come to recognize that it may be as important to model scientific communication across disciplinary boundaries as it is to train students to become interdisciplinarians themselves. Indeed the most versatile biomedical scientist of the future may be the individual who can reach across disciplines and inspire collaboration among those with different training and expertise. We believe that the most effective way to inspire and galvanize interest in key correlative disciplines is through the laboratory. By discovering the motivation for utilizing approaches from other disciplines, biology students see these fields as live and vital. In addition, they also become confident in their ability to learn new areas of science that might—as dictated by their experiments—be relevant to their research throughout their career. Notably, they view this process as collaborative, and they become comfortable seeing themselves as learners who evolve in intellectual conversation with computer scientists, physicists, mathematicians, and chemists. And of course faculty satisfaction and research productivity are also often much higher when the process is thoughtfully interactive.

For these reasons we find two parallel approaches effective. First, we see the benefits of recommending (and in some cases requiring) that students in biology study chemistry, physics, computer science, and/or mathematics at an advanced level. Recommendations vary depending on the interests of the student, but we stress the importance of specific relevant areas of competency. Second, in our intermediate and upper-level laboratory experimental work we try to pick topics that utilize and integrate these related disciplines (e.g., the mathematical foundations of computational genomics, the physics of fluorescence-activated cell sorters, and the chemistry of small molecule compound modification from chemical libraries). Ideally these laboratories are designed collaboratively between members of different departments and are sometimes team-taught. Assignments in other courses often emphasize problems that require students to consult information and individuals outside their major.

As with the laboratory experience, the students can also see interdisciplinary investigation modeled in the activities of the faculty members. Liberal arts colleges have a great advantage for training in interdisciplinary sciences in that students and faculty members interact easily and often across traditional departmental boundaries—both formally and informally. The students expect that they, like the faculty members they observe, will have productive and collegial relationships with faculty members in many other scientific disciplines.

In fact many students enter college with a natural ease in interdisciplinary studies. They have been taking biology, chemistry, and math courses in high school and do not perceive the integration of mathematics with biology or other sciences to be unusual. The challenge for the faculty members is not to persuade students that interdisciplinary studies are important but rather to encourage and develop further the appropriate integration of interdisciplinary sciences in the curriculum. Ultimately our seniors will have spent three years growing increasingly comfortable working as independent experimenters who function in an interdisciplinary team environment. They expect to work in such environments in graduate school and beyond.

Students Should Become Comfortable Communicating Science

All working biomedical investigators know the importance of communicating their work in manuscripts, posters, presentations, grant applications, and orally, in both hallways and conference halls. The ability to articulate clearly the purpose and approach of an experimental endeavor and to engage in discourse about scientific advances is invaluable, and makes participation in the scientific community both possible and truly enjoyable. Without these communication skills, laboratory work becomes an isolated, uphill struggle. Perhaps that is why a surprising number of our nation's most successful biomedical investigators were not undergraduate biology or chemistry majors but English majors. Whatever the undergraduate concentration, however, the ability to develop scientific narratives orally and in writing is paramount, and the liberal arts setting is an ideal place to refine these academic virtues.

In the context of undergraduate science education, faculty can work to encourage their students to communicate clearly, effectively, and frequently. The classic importance of clear exposition in the laboratory notebook has not changed or diminished. But there are now many additional activities that are more incisively targeted at community involvement and communication, including participation in laboratory meetings and critical journal clubs, preparation and delivery of public presentations at all levels of the curriculum, construction of posters and their live presentation at poster sessions, and writing mock grant proposals as course assignments. Most worthwhile are opportunities for undergraduates to participate in regional and national scientific meetings by communicating their own work through oral or poster formats. In these settings, students must hone their communication skills while simultaneously getting immediate positive feedback for their participation in the scientific community.

Summary

The foregoing analysis describes one historically successful approach to modeling, inspiring, and training undergraduate students for future careers in biomedical investigation. Of course there is no one formula for developing the abilities and passion for biomedical research that define nascent physician-scientists. Nevertheless, any curriculum that intentionally exposes students to problem-solving approaches in multiple disciplines, that requires students to develop a scholarly expertise so they may gain ownership of an issue and gain entry into a community of scholarship, and encourages them to explore or "play" with ideas as they work toward solutions will go a long way toward developing students who will be both inspired and empowered to take on the challenges of any research career. Fundamentally, the more we model science as an activity whose joys and satisfactions are seen continuously in its pursuit, the stronger and more resilient will be the pipeline of future biomedical investigators.

8

The Role of Academic Medical Centers and Medical Schools in the Training and Support of Physician-Scientists

Philip A. Pizzo, MD

The education, training, and career development of physician-scientists has evolved in parallel with the sweeping changes in medicine that have occurred in the United States beginning in the post–Civil War era. As described in chapter 1 by Andrew Schafer, in the last half of the nineteenth century, medical education was largely devoid of a scientific tradition or foundation. Physicians interested in research traveled to Europe (especially Germany, Italy, and France) to pursue their training and career goals. In the 1880s Charles Eliot of Harvard, along with the presidents of several other public and private universities, began a reformation of medical education that introduced science into the curriculum, and the first academic medical centers (AMCs) began to emerge.

Some of the AMCs developed as alignments between existing universities, medical schools, and hospitals, whereas others, such as Johns Hopkins, were founded on the three pillars that have long defined the repertoire of the physician-scientist: teaching, research, and patient care. A more formalized introduction of science into medical education followed the Flexner Report of 1910. Over the first half of the twentieth century, a number of AMCs began to focus on the important role that physician-scientists play in the evolution of knowledge and the care of patients. But in many ways AMCs as we know them today are really a product of the second half of the twentieth century. They were shaped by—and responsive to—the then new and increasing funding for research from the National Institutes of

Health following the 1944 Public Health Service Act, which initiated the NIH research grants program.

From the 1960s until the late 1980s and early 1990s, most AMCs flourished by expanding their faculty, constructing new and larger research facilities, and increasing the size and complexity of their clinical enterprises. A renewed emphasis on research faculty and facilities again emerged during and in anticipation of the doubling of the NIH budget between 1998 and 2003. This expansion, however, has since run into difficulty because of the declining support for biomedical research from the NIH that has occurred since 2003.

Initially, few AMCs had sufficient depth and expertise in basic and clinical science, and the tradition of sending promising physician-scientists to train in the Intramural Program of the National Institutes of Health became the norm. These young physician-scientists, equipped with new knowledge and expertise, were then recruited back to universities, medical schools, and teaching hospitals, where they founded and expanded new research programs supported by peer-reviewed funding from the extramural grants programs of the NIH. Eventually the vector toward Bethesda reversed toward the leading research-intensive AMCs. In these institutions newly minted physician-scientists helped redefine medical education, academic research, and changes in patient care. The synergy worked, since the direct and indirect funding provided by the NIH helped to recruit the faculty and develop research-intensive clinical departments as well as strong basic science departments. Furthermore, the clinical surpluses associated with "fee-for-service" clinical medicine, buffered by federal entitlement programs such as Medicare and Medicaid, permitted teaching hospitals to grow and expand and to use surplus financial earnings to reinvest in education, research, and facilities.

Not unexpectedly, the dynamics of these changes affected AMCs differently, with stronger programs for research more likely to take place at universities and medical schools that were traditionally oriented toward research. The growth in biomedical research, fueled largely by the NIH, permitted a number of medical schools, universities, and teaching hospitals to intensify and expand their research base significantly, often with transformational institutional consequences. The extraordinary discoveries that have occurred across the domains of basic and clinical science during the past half century further catalyzed this process. This has resulted in the emergence of new disciplines, the creation of new tools and technologies to support and enhance inquiry and investigation, as well as the development of vast databases and the powerful tools needed for their collection, storage, and analysis. The ever-increasing complexity and sophistication of science and the regulatory and compliance forces that oversee discovery and, especially, human subjects research have also been part of this process.

All of this has further resulted in either the increased integration of the AMC into the fabric of the university or, in some cases, its separation into discrete entities. It has also led to important connections with industry to support research and translate knowledge from the laboratory to the patient. On the one hand, greater interdependency between academic institutions and industry has resulted in sometimes troubling individual and institutional conflicts of interest. On the other hand, it has created centers of excellence in biomedical research that are unsurpassed in the world. Finally, we now find that there are enormous vulnerabilities when the funding streams and sources change or decline or when the landscape for medical care or research is subject to local, regional, or national shifts in support.

Evolving Market Forces and Academic Medicine

Many of the notable changes that have occurred in AMCs have been the consequence of market forces. When the fee-for-service platform moved to a market-driven managed care environment in the early 1990s, significant changes in the landscape of AMCs soon followed. As the clinical profit margins fell dramatically, the demands for increased patient throughput and greater efficiencies led AMCs to establish new expectations for faculty physician patient care workloads. When this occurred, it decreased the time that physician-scientists who had limited NIH funding could devote to research, compelling them to increase their clinical time and, as a consequence, decrease their opportunity for academic productivity. This challenge was particularly pronounced for junior faculty, whose limited research funding led their department chairs to direct them to take on additional clinical care responsibilities. While this challenge has been difficult for all faculty, it has been especially so for women, whose academic careers are particularly impacted by their attempts to balance work and family pressures.

Since the early 1990s the dynamics between providers (physicians and other health care professionals) and the hospitals or clinics where they carry out their work have been increasingly counterpoised to those of the payers (whether the insurance industry or government entitlement programs). This has led hospital leaders and their overseers to seek new organizational models (e.g., mergers, primary care networks, various physician-hospital organizations) to ensure (or increase) financial performance. Clearly the extent to which financial performance becomes a dominant institutional goal has significant implications for sustaining an environment that fosters the training, career development, and success of physician-scientists. Over time a number of institutions have tilted more strongly toward their patient care than their research mission. As a consequence their success in attracting or developing physician-scientists has declined or has become threatened.

Just as the financial pressures on teaching hospitals can shift the focus, commitment, and support away from basic and clinical research, so too can changes in the support for research from the NIH. While the United States cannot boast a health care system that is a model of excellence, efficiency, and success, that is not the case for biomedical research. Indeed the investments in research from the NIH, National Science Foundation, and numerous private not-for-profit foundations, as well as industry and individual philanthropists, have made bioscience in the United States the best in the world. And while there have been ups and downs in the funding for biomedical research, none has been as dramatic as what has taken place since the late 1990s. In 1998, with broad bipartisan congressional support, the NIH began the doubling of its budget (from $13 billion to $26 billion). This doubling was also the product of public recognition that new opportunities to advance knowledge or to impact the outcome of human disease would be stimulated by vigorous research.

It was broadly believed that additional funding would encourage more physicians to engage in research and that this might also stimulate more PhD scientists to consider translational in addition to fundamental research. Support for the doubling of NIH funding came from academic leaders, professional societies, and disease advocacy groups, and was actualized by champions of the NIH within Congress, notably Congressman John Porter (R-Ill.), Senator Arlen Specter (R-Pa.), and Senator Ted Kennedy (D-Mass.), among others. The doubling of the NIH budget, which was completed in 2003, was accompanied by a number of events that promoted the recruitment, development, and sustenance of physician-scientists at AMCs. This is measured by a significant increase in the number of individuals who succeeded in receiving peer-reviewed NIH funding—creating a sense of hope and promise within academic communities and especially among junior physician-scientists—as well as students, residents, and fellows aspiring to join their ranks. This was accompanied by institutional decisions to expand programs and facilities to support the research mission of AMCs. Many AMC leaders assumed that the doubling of the NIH budget would be sustained and thus rushed to construct new research facilities to support and recruit faculty for what was envisioned to be an enlarging research mission. While many well-established AMCs joined this bandwagon, so too did new AMCs or those whose research mission had been marginal. By making major capital and program investments and commitments, many AMCs became vulnerable to generating a nonsustainable capacity for biomedical research.

For a variety of reasons (among them too many promises about how increased funding would lead to cures of major diseases; somewhat naïve expectations in the public and private sectors as to when a "return on investment" would be evident; tensions within universities over the disproportionate funding for biomedical as compared to physical science research; and unanticipated dramatic changes in the U.S. economy from a surplus to a large deficit), NIH support was not sustained, even at the rate of inflation, after the doubling. Instead the NIH budget remained flat and below inflation with a greater than 13 percent decline in purchasing power.

At this writing the serious economic events that reached global proportions beginning in September–October 2008 make it likely that improvements in NIH funding, even at levels that keep pace with inflation, are now more questionable. This has created enormous consequences and pressures in AMCs in general and for physician-scientists in particular. Competition for funding has increased enormously, success rates for NIH grant applications have fallen (to below 10 percent), the need to write more grants has consumed more and more time, institutional overhead for excess space has become more difficult to achieve, and the general morale in academic medical centers has declined. The pressures for success and the need to balance the tripartite missions of teaching, research, and patient care are difficult enough. Coupled with the increasing pressures of faculty seeking to find balance in their personal and professional lives or to meet the pressures of a national economic downturn, they have become even more significant.

While there seems no end in sight, with most knowledgeable individuals anticipating that federal support for biomedical research is likely to remain below inflation for at least a period of several years, this has been ameliorated through 2011 because of $10.4 billion of funding for science included in the economic stimulus plan formulated by the Obama administration as part of the American Recovery and Reinvestment Act (ARRA) of 2009. Whether funding will be sustained, and at what level, once the ARRA has run its course at the end of 2010 remains to be seen and will be surely impacted by the fragility of the U.S. economy.

Thus the role of AMCs in supporting and developing physician-scientists has been influenced not only by institutional resources and commitment but also by external forces—especially those that impact the funding profiles for teaching hospitals and the research mission. When these forces are out of sync, they can tilt some AMCs to move in a direction they might not have planned for or chosen. When they occur in tandem—as they will likely continue to do for some years to come—the results could be far-reaching. An AMC's ability to sustain a commitment to educating and supporting physician-scientists will be influenced not only by the vision and commitment of its leaders and the excellence of its faculty, students, and staff but also by its ability to overcome the external funding challenges.

Organization and Governance of AMCs and Their Impact on the Education, Training, and Development of Physician-Scientists

Among the approximately 125 medical schools and academic medical centers in the United States, there are numerous models of organization and governance as well as missions. These result in variations in the balance of focus, emphasis, and support for education, research, and patient care. Some of these AMCs are known as "research-intensive," often measured by the amount of NIH funding for research or the percentage or number of faculty engaged in research. Others are referred to as "primary care" medical schools, largely because of their greater focus on patient care and clinical teaching than on basic and clinical research. Depending on their size, complexity, and available resources, some are able to support significant research as well as primary care missions. That said, each is challenged when the external resources and funding to support either the clinical or the research mission become constrained. The depth and breadth of research-oriented faculty, available resources, and institutional culture can influence the decision of a medical student to pursue a career as a physician-scientist—or not. Nevertheless, highly motivated students can emerge as future physician-scientists from centers where resources are limited and the focus is not on research, just as students in resource-rich research environments may elect to pursue a pathway distinctly different from that of a physician-scientist.

The organizational models for AMCs and their relative focus on research or patient care are often historically derived. Some AMCs include a constellation of health profession schools (medicine, dentistry, nursing, pharmacy, public health) along with teaching hospitals, whereas others include one or more professional schools with various types of hospital affiliations. The affiliated teaching hospitals either are "owned" by the medical school or parent university or are independent and enjoined through an affiliation agreement. Faculty (including physician-scientists) can be employed by the medical school or university, the teaching hospital, or a separate foundation or physician group (or practice plan). Notably, most AMCs are physically separated from their parent university. The affiliated teaching hospitals may be proximate to or distant from the research facilities of an AMC. In a smaller number of cases the medical school and affiliated teaching hospitals are contiguous to each other and, on occasion, to the parent university as well. Both the geographic as well as organizational configurations have an impact on how an AMC functions and how it supports current and future physician-scientists.

The governance of AMCs is also highly varied. Some have a single leader with oversight over the medical and other health professional schools as well as teaching hospitals, whereas others have separate leaders for medical and professional schools as well as teaching hospitals. Furthermore, some teaching hospitals are led by physician administrators (who potentially may be more attentive to the importance of physician-scientists), whereas others are led by professional hospital administrators. Regardless of the governance structure or background credentials of the leadership, the ability to align resources to support the missions of education, research, and patient care depends on the willingness and ability of leaders to work collaboratively and to enunciate and implement a shared mission. Clearly this can change over time. The availability of external resources and funding that support the financial viability of the teaching hospital and/or medical school also influences the alignment of their missions. When external resources become challenged, the commitment of the leaders and the internal resources (endowment, reserves, philanthropic support) become essential ingredients for success.

Given the wide array of organization and governance among AMCs, it is hard to conclude that any single model is the most successful—or even if successful, that it is sustainable over time in fostering the career development of physician-scientists. Moreover, as noted, successful physician-scientists can emerge from AMCs whose mission is to develop them—or from those that have different orientations. For example, the Johns Hopkins University School of Medicine, one of the best in the world, was founded as an integrated teaching hospital and medical school. It has a long tradition of honoring excellence in patient care as well as research and an exemplary record of educating and developing academically oriented physicians. Hopkins Medicine is physically separated from its parent university and is also unique in that it dwarfs the university in its relative size and resources. While its governance has changed over time, at this writing its executive dean is responsible for both the medical school and its teaching hospital. This model of integration has been successful in aligning the missions of education, research, and patient care. Yet very different models also are highly successful.

Harvard Medicine also has a long historical tradition as well as one of the more unusual models—but also with a remarkable record of educating and developing an extraordinary array of leaders in academic medicine and the biosciences. Harvard Medicine comprises schools of medicine, dentistry, and public health, each separately governed and physically separated from its parent university. It is also unique in that its major teaching hospitals all have distinguished records in their own right, as well as large endowments. Harvard's hospitals include the Massachusetts General Hospital (MGH), Brigham and Women's Hospital, and the Dana-Farber Cancer Center, which form the nucleus of Partners Healthcare; the Beth Israel and New England Deaconess Hospitals, which constitute the merged CareGroup; and the Children's Hospital, Boston, which stands independently. These hospitals also employ both physicians and basic scientists, and manage their own research, education, and patient care missions. In the aggregate Harvard Medicine is the largest in the nation, with over eight thousand full-time faculty, most of whom reside in one of the affiliated teaching hospitals. Not only are these faculty responsible for clinical teaching, but also many are engaged in teaching the medical school's preclinical curriculum. Each of the major hospitals has a basic science faculty which in itself matches those of other research-intensive medical schools in size and excellence. Although physicians lead each of these entities (the medical school and major affiliated teaching hospitals), they are also autonomous and only loosely connected to the others and to the medical school. Harvard Medicine has a remarkably strong history in research, education, and patient care and has been one of the most successful institutions in the world in educating, developing, and supporting physician-scientists. That said, the challenges of managed care have had a notably deleterious impact on the ability of the teaching hospitals to work collaboratively, and in fact have often led them into direct competition.

Institutional leaders and external or internal forces can, clearly, positively and sometimes negatively influence a commitment or recommitment to the education and development of physician-scientists. For example, the University of Pittsburgh School of Medicine has accrued considerable resources from its parent hospital system and from the allocation of the state tobacco tax. These resources, coupled with the commitment of institutional leadership, focused the medical student curriculum on the education of academic physicians. On a different scale, when the Cleveland

Clinic decided to launch a small medical school, it was clear in delineating its purpose of educating future physician-scientists. This is in contrast to the medical school being developed at the University of California, Merced, where the focus is on educating physicians who will be more engaged in rural care. Without question it is helpful for medical schools to make their mission clear so that students can better appreciate the institutional goals, thus better ensuring the success and satisfaction of both students and faculty.

Stanford as an Example

Many of the challenges and opportunities in educating, training, and supporting physician-scientists can be appreciated by examining the Stanford experience. In a number of ways it exemplifies, albeit on a smaller scale, how institutional focus can be directed to—or diverted from—a commitment to physician-scientists. In relating some of the past history and current events, I do not wish to convey that past or current models are better or worse; rather I mean to show how they can create environments and cultures that enhance or detract from the future of academically oriented physicians.

Stanford Medical School has had two beginnings. The first was in 1908, when Stanford University (then only seventeen years old) assimilated the Cooper Medical College (which dated back to 1858) to become the Stanford University School of Medicine. At that time, however, and for the subsequent fifty years, the clinical locus of the medical school was in San Francisco, some thirty-five miles north of the Palo Alto campus that houses Stanford University. Although a number of faculty were engaged in research, for the first half century of its existence Stanford Medical School was largely a regional and clinically oriented institution. In the early to mid-1950s a faculty report aligned with the vision of the university president (a historian) and provost (an engineer) of Stanford. They both recognized that the second half of the twentieth century and beyond would give birth to a revolution in human biology and medicine and that Stanford University—as well as the medical school—would benefit by locating the medical school on the university campus. In 1959 Stanford Medical School moved to the Stanford campus. It now adjoins the school of engineering and the buildings housing the biological and physical sciences at the university, as well as its two major affiliated teaching hospitals. This physical contiguity has so far proved critical in shaping Stanford Medicine—and also in advancing the university as a research powerhouse.

A number of factors converged to shape the early development of Stanford Medicine, some of which persist today. Perhaps most notable was the decision to create new departments (initially biochemistry and genetics) and to recruit outstanding individuals to lead them. Almost single-handedly this shaped the second (post-1959) phase of the medical school as an institution committed to science and the development of physician-scientists. Specifically, Arthur Kornberg, MD, was recruited from Washington University, where he was chair of microbiology, to lead a new department of biochemistry at Stanford. One of his conditions for moving to Stanford was that he be able to bring with him his entire department from Washington University—which he did. The five individuals who accompanied him went on to have extraordinarily distinguished careers individually, and formed the nucleus and focus of the "new" medical school by anchoring it in a deep commitment to innovative basic science, a tradition that continues to this day. This was enhanced when Dr. Kornberg won the Nobel Prize in Medicine shortly after his arrival at Stanford. His own deep commitment to the close linkage of science and medicine in both research and education also fueled the school's mission. Soon after his own arrival, Kornberg and others recruited Dr. Joshua Lederberg from the University of Wisconsin to found a new department of genetics at Stanford. He too soon had a Nobel Prize, and the landscape of Stanford Medicine was rapidly changed from a clinical to a research focus.

This transition was impacted by the fact that many of the prominent clinical leaders and department chairs of the medical school located in San Francisco elected not to make the move, since Palo Alto was seen as quite remote from the thriving clinical practices they had in the city. There were a couple of notable exceptions, however. Henry Kaplan came as chair of radiology and became one of the fathers of radiation oncology, joining forces with Edward Ginzton from the physics department to develop the first linear accelerator used in clinical medicine. This important intersection of science and medicine laid the foundation for fostering a culture of interdisciplinary research, another facet of Stanford that characterizes its past and present. Avrum Goldstein also moved from San Francisco to Palo Alto and laid the foundations for the future of pharmacology. Dr. Norm Shumway, then quite junior, likewise made the move and forged new relationships between surgery and immunology to develop cardiac transplant biology, leading to the first heart transplant in the United States and the foundations of excellence in the new field of cardiovascular surgery and research. Outstanding physician-scientist leaders in medicine, pediatrics, and psychiatry, among other disciplines, soon joined this core group of faculty leaders and collectively created a vibrant environment in which to educate and train physician-scientists. This was coupled with a novel education program called "The Five Year Plan," denoting the fact that all medical students would spend at least an additional year in medical school, and each would combine research with the medical school curriculum. Because the vision and goal of the medical school was clearly defined, it attracted students who shared an interest in research—many of whom became committed to careers as physician-scientists and now serve as leaders at academic medical centers across the United States and around the world.

At the same time, the focus on science, and especially basic science, was so strong that it became the metric for institutional success, and in some ways the perceived standard for success at Stanford. An inadvertent consequence was that an equal respect for clinical medicine was not as deeply fostered. Stanford became so oriented toward research that clinical medicine developed more episodically and did not hold the same esteem in the eyes of a number of the faculty. Whereas at some institutions being an outstanding clinician is on equal footing to being a scientist, this was not the case at Stanford during the first years of its move to Palo Alto.

While the focus of Stanford remained closely aligned to basic research, the students who entered in the early 1970s felt increasingly disenfranchised and sought more engagement in community activities rather than time in the laboratory. The medical school curriculum evolved to become more flexible and, as an inadvertent consequence, less clear in defining an institutional value or career path for incoming students. Once again, in the mid- to late 1990s outside influences distracted the medical center as a whole when the Stanford Medical Center merged with—and then demerged from—the University of California, San Francisco (UCSF). These events serve to point out that in an environment otherwise fertile for their education, both internal and external forces can redirect the training of physician-scientists.

Although educating and training physician-scientists was still very much part of the fabric and culture of Stanford when I arrived as dean in April 2001, it had lost some of its original focus. The medical education curriculum had not been revised for some time. It did, however, contain an important program called "Medical Scholars" that permitted students to carry out research and scholarship in selected areas. More important was the need to rebuild the alignment between the basic and clinical science faculty and between the medical center and the university—both of which had become challenged during the failed merger attempt with UCSF. That said, the fundamental building blocks were in place to refocus the education and training programs. Most important was the overall excellence of the basic science faculty, the physical contiguity of the school to the university, the excellence of the students and trainees, and a willingness of each to move in new directions—including returning to core principles.

Upon my arrival as dean, Stanford Medical School began a comprehensive strategic planning program which continues to this day and which commenced with a redefinition of mission: *"To be a premier research-intensive medical school that improves health through leadership and collaborative discoveries and innovation in patient care, education and research."* In accord with a proposal for transformation that I announced on my first day at Stanford, work groups were assembled to assess and then address integrated planning in undergraduate medical student education, graduate education, resident and postdoctoral training, basic and clinical research, the focus of patient care activities, the composition and evolution of the professoriate, the financial and administrative infrastructure necessary to support core missions in education, research, and clinical care, the enhancement of communication strategies, development of advocacy programs to support core missions, and the construction of the machinery to develop fundraising and philanthropy to support core programmatic initiatives and new facilities. To move these agendas forward, an office of institutional planning was established and regular updates of progress were presented to the school's Executive Committee (composed of basic and clinical science chairs, institute directors, and senior decanal leaders) as well as in my biweekly "Dean's Newsletter," available online. In addition, progress reports and planning for future initiatives occur each year at the Medical School Leadership Retreat.

An important aspect of the strategic planning efforts has been aligning core missions in education, research, and patient care. As a small research-intensive school of medicine, we determined to focus our educational programs on educating and developing future physician-scientists and scholars and in highlighting opportunities to "translate discoveries." This has resulted in the construction of a new curriculum for medical student education that requires every student to engage in a scholarly concentration that involves research. It also includes efforts to better align medical education across the continuum of learning from undergraduate through graduate medical education with opportunities for joint degree programs for medical students and advanced residents or clinical fellows. In parallel, it involves programs permitting graduate students to learn about clinical medicine and translational research through a master's in medical science degree.

Stanford has a long history of graduates who pursue full-time careers in academic medicine. Best estimates suggest that approximately 30 percent of graduating MD students are in academic medicine full-time, as physician-scientists, clinician-scholars, or clinician educators. A goal of our New Stanford Curriculum is to increase the number of graduates pursuing careers in academic medicine to 50 percent or more. This requires better aligning the curriculum with the career goals and aspirations of the students who are selected for admission to Stanford. Indeed it is now widely appreciated that with the New Curriculum, students coming to Stanford are more focused on research and scholarship than when a more flexible curriculum existed and an institutional focus was not as clearly enunciated.

The key components of the New Curriculum include a close connection between science and medicine throughout medical school. This means that students are introduced to clinical medicine at the same time they are learning the foundations of molecular medicine, organ systems, and disease. It also means that students on clinical clerkships have opportunities for science-based correlations with the illnesses and problems they are encountering.

A key and unique feature of the New Stanford Curriculum, which was introduced in the fall of 2003, was a requirement that every student pursue a scholarly concentration. To enable students to engage in focused areas of research and scholarship, it was necessary to make time in the curriculum. Two steps were taken to accomplish this: first, didactic courses were each cut back by approximately 25 percent. This resulted in one day per week without scheduled classes during the first quarter and then subsequently up to two free days per week for independent scholarship. Students can choose from a wide range of scholarly concentrations—including bioethics and the humanities, bioengineering, bio-computation, community health and public service, health policy, molecular medicine, clinical research, and more. Each scholarly concentration has a core faculty, prescribed courses, and opportunities for research. If none of the available scholarly concentrations meets the student's interests, an independent concentration can be established.

A second key facet of the Stanford Medicine education is that approximately three-quarters of students do five or more years of medical school—further increasing their time for research and scholarly pursuits. Because of Stanford's tuition assistance programs, students graduate with among the lowest levels of indebtedness among both public and private schools, even with the extra years of medical school. This additional time is important in permitting students to develop experience in research and academics and thus is strongly encouraged. Since, however, a number of students come to Stanford with an advanced degree or extensive prior research experience or begin their studies later in life, we have elected not to mandate a required five-year program but rather refer to it as a "flexible five-year program."

The New Stanford Curriculum also provides opportunities for students to earn joint degrees at the master's or PhD level. Joint degree opportunities now exist with each Stanford school (Engineering, Humanities and Sciences, Education, Business, Law, Earth Sciences) and we have students who are in fact pursuing such degrees throughout the university. These joint degree opportunities complement the traditional MSTP (medical scientist training program; see chapter 9 by Roy Silverstein and Paul DiCorleto), which has existed at Stanford for some forty years and which has a high level of success. Recognizing that a number of students do not develop their desire for a combined MD-PhD degree until after they begin medical school and a scholarly concentration, we now admit an equal number of students to an MSTP track after they have gained entrance to the medical school. Notably, the number of students deciding to pursue MD-PhD studies has increased since the introduction of the New Curriculum.

An important but still unfulfilled goal is to improve the alignment of education and training from undergraduate through graduate medical education (see chapter 7 by Stephen Emerson, Philip Meneely, and Jennifer Punt). Efforts are under way to do this, but much work remains. At the same time, we have introduced a program for advanced residents or clinical fellows who become interested in careers as physician-scientists. This program—known as Advanced Residency Training at Stanford (ARTS)—permits selected residents and fellows to pursue a PhD degree while completing their clinical training. Institutional support is provided to cover both the stipend and tuition, making it an attractive option for "late-blooming" physician-scientists. We believe, as does Kenneth Kaushansky (see chapter 10), that this is an important group of individuals since they are even more likely to continue their work as physician-scientists. This program has already supported trainees from surgical disciplines as well as the more traditional medical ones.

In summary, we have refocused our institutional efforts on educating and training physician-scientists and scholars from undergraduate through graduate medical education. In doing so, we are attracting students and trainees who are aligned with our programmatic directions. It remains to be seen, however, whether these programs and opportunities will increase the number of our graduates who pursue academic careers and whether they will make them more successful should they choose this career pathway. Clearly, in addition to the goals and ambitions of our students and trainees, important institutional and broader societal and economic forces impact the potential for success.

The Next Phase in the Career Path of Physician-Scientists

In addition to enlarging the pipeline of future physician-scientists, equally if not more important is the role that AMCs play in supporting career development. This often means the amount of institutional support that is provided to launch a career, the amount of protected time made available for research, the mentoring and career development support that is provided, the institutional culture, and clarity of the appointment and promotion systems that are in place. The last is especially relevant to faculty who pursue clinical and translational research where team-based research is more the norm.

Virtually all U.S. medical schools have developed along a model of leveraged federal support. That is, research is largely funded by the NIH or other federal agencies through a competitive peer review process. The model for reviewing basic science research faculty is well established—as are the criteria for appointment and promotion in most medical schools and universities. Less well established are the sources of support for clinical research, especially for those engaged in clinical trials research. Equally, the criteria for appointment and promotion are more challenging since the length of time required for clinical research to reach fruition is relatively long and is often team-based, making the identification of unique individual contributions difficult to establish. While most academic centers recognize the importance of stratifying career paths and promotion requirements, it still remains a challenge for faculty who are trying to split their time between clinical and research work. Ultimately it is a matter of balance, expectations, institutional commitment, and careful mentoring.

Most AMCs, including Stanford, have developed different academic tracks that are relevant for physician-scientists. At Stanford we have three major tracks, and physician-scientists generally reside in two of these: the investigator track, which assumes that at least 80 percent of faculty time is spent in research, and the clinician-scholar/clinician-investigator track, with 40–60 percent (on average) of time in research or patient care activities, respectively. Physician-scientists can fit into either track. In the investigator track it is expected that the faculty member will be successful in securing funding from peer-reviewed sources and that clinical income will represent a minor source of support. Moreover, appointment and promotion for investigators are based on the quality and impact of independent research contributions. Physician-scientists in the investigator track can reside in either basic or clinical science departments.

In contrast, if a faculty member is in the clinician-investigator/clinician-scholar track, the sources of support are proportional to the time spent in either patient care or research activities. These faculty members serve as the critical bridge between basic and clinical science and are instrumental in facilitating and conducting translational and clinical research. But they require careful mentoring and protection. Unfortunately, in most AMCs they are often caught in the crosscurrents between expectations for heightened clinical productivity and those regarding the mix and quality of research and teaching contributions. While many faculty desire to blend research with patient care activities, they face a significant degree of institutional vulnerability and stress as they try to balance different goals and objectives to meet sometimes divergent standards and expectations.

While all clinician-investigators/clinician-scholars face similar ambiguities of institutional commitment and expectation, the challenge is even greater for women, who are often also balancing professional and personal demands—frequently including a disproportionate share of family responsibilities. I recently had the opportunity to meet with each junior faculty woman at Stanford. While there were large differences in how individuals were facing the challenges of career development, it was clear that success was most likely when the division or department they were in was attentive and responsive to their needs and where thoughtful mentoring and career advice were provided. Clearly this varies among AMCs and also within an academic institution.

Although it is easy to point to the success stories of physician-scientists in AMCs, it is more important to focus on the failures and adversities. It should be a safe assumption that each faculty appointment has the prospect for success. It is important to recognize, however, that internal and external events and pressures can conspire against success. In some cases there is a breach of understanding between the junior faculty member and her or his immediate supervisor or department chair. This can involve differences in the expectations for external funding, time spent on clinical service, and research and/or clinical productivity. Changes in institutional leadership or support (including from the hospital), as well as changes in the external funding environment, can pose additional problems. Notably these factors and issues can vary among different departments or programs within a single AMC as well as among them. Many junior faculty members feel uninformed about the expectations or criteria on which their performance will be judged, and all too often there is an incomplete or inadequate sharing of career advice by senior faculty or department chairs. This is especially true when the performance of a faculty member is less than optimal, and where there is an unfortunate reluctance to offer candid, transparent, and direct advice—even if painfully delivered or received.

It is also important to underscore that the focus and commitment of an AMC for physician-scientists extend throughout the career pathway—from junior to mid-career and senior faculty status. The issues and challenges that arise are different, but certain common themes can be defined. These include the availability of institutional support to bridge loss of grant support, the value placed on academic pursuits versus clinical productivity, the criteria used to assess promotion, and the presence of mentors and career advisers skilled in the various stages of development of a physician-scientist.

Some Observations and Lessons Learned

- Academic medical centers play a critical role in the education, training, support, and success or failure of physician-scientists. Many factors contribute to successful or unsuccessful outcomes—some controllable but other aspects more subjective and less controllable.
- It is possible to construct curricula and an institutional culture that selects and then nurtures students who aspire to become physician-scientists and scholars. Nevertheless, continuing support through the continuum of undergraduate and graduate medical education and into junior and more senior faculty appointments is challenging. In part this is because oversight of different phases of training, education, and career development falls under the province of different programs and leaders in an AMC, not all of which are aligned in their priorities and mission. There is a need to develop training paths that are integrated across the education and training domains and continue through faculty appointment and subsequent career development.
- Not all medical schools or institutions are equipped or able to train, educate, and support physician-scientists. While there may be a sense that this should be expected of every medical school and AMC, the stark reality is that the institutional resources, commitments, and values vary considerably, and as a consequence, so do the outcomes and successes.
- Evidence of institutional commitment is essential at the time of recruitment and appointment of a junior faculty physician-scientist and is evidenced by the size and scope of the recruitment package. Failure to provide the resources needed to launch a career path is a prescription for failure. So too is a lack of continued mentoring, guidance, and candid career development advice.

- Institutional culture and expectations play an important role in defining and delineating career pathways, avenues for success, the criteria and requirements for appointment and promotions. The institutional culture can be influenced by the attitudes and actions of leaders within the university, medical school, teaching hospitals, and community.
- External forces, particularly the funding for research or demands for clinical service, can impact success and influence the pipeline for developing new physician-scientists. The current economic climate poses serious challenges and, if extended, could undermine the primacy of the United States as a leader in biomedical research.
- Despite the challenges, a career as a physician-scientist and scholar is filled with wonder, excitement, opportunity, relevance, and impact. It is certainly a career pathway I have much enjoyed and would encourage others to follow.

9

The Relationship between Physicians and PhD Scientists in Medical Research

Roy L. Silverstein, MD, and Paul E. DiCorleto, PhD

Only a small number of individuals have been charged with directing the National Institutes of Health (NIH) during its modern era, and each has left behind an important legacy. One of the significant accomplishments of Dr. Elias Zerhouni, director of the NIH from 2002 to 2008, was to awaken the scientific, government, and lay communities to the large gap that exists between research progress at the laboratory bench and its impact in the clinic. The once rarely heard term "translational research"—that is, research designed to bridge that gap—has now become a common phrase in the scientific lexicon, appearing on the covers of major journals and in the names of new academic departments and centers. The genesis of this gap lies in the turbocharged expansion of basic and disease-oriented laboratory research precipitated by the molecular revolution during an era that paradoxically saw dramatic shrinking in the relative numbers of patient-oriented clinical researchers. In the years since James Wyngaarden wrote famously of the "demise" of the physician-scientist (Wyngaarden 1979), the situation has only gotten worse. In 1970 the ratio of investigator-initiated NIH grants awarded to physician researchers versus PhD investigators was approximately 50:50, compared to 20:80 in 2008 (Butler 2008).

The shortage of clinical researchers has been attributed to several factors (Goldstein and Brown 1997), including the regulatory and financial burdens faced by practicing physicians and academic clinical departments, which make it very difficult to do clinical research while practicing medicine. Among other contributors to the decline are the retreat from clinical and translational research by Big Pharma, due at least partly to economic considerations; the inability of the time-restricted medical school preclinical curriculum to keep up with the growing complexity of modern science; the increasingly hostile funding and regulatory environment for clinical research; the NIH salary cap, which is set substantially lower than the actual salaries of many medical and surgical subspecialists; and the emergence of clinical research fields that some have considered "nontranslational" (see the introduction to this book), such as health services research, as alternatives for physicians interested in an investigative career. In this context it is useful to examine the relationship between physician and nonphysician researchers, particularly those with PhDs, and to consider how this relationship can be expanded and exploited to advance the needs of effective translational research. That there is room to improve this relationship is not contested. In fact Barbara Alving, a physician hematologist and director of the NIH's National Center for Research Resources (the funding agency for the now defunct General Clinical Research Center program and its successor, the Clinical Translational Science Award program), has been quoted as stating that "clinical and basic scientists don't really communicate" (Butler 2008).

Early History of MD-PhD Interactions

As further explored in chapter 1 by Andrew Schafer, the history of modern biomedical investigation can be traced to the early twentieth century, when the Flexner Report in 1910 led to a reorganization of American medical education into an "academic" model based on science, research, and scholarship rather than apprenticeship. The period between the Flexner Report and the first few years after the Second World War was marked by the emergence of academic medical centers, exemplified by those located at well-established private universities and their affiliated hospitals in the cities of the East and Midwest, as well as those at the larger research-centered state universities, mostly in the Midwest. During this era medical students were taught the "preclinical" curriculum of anatomy, physiology, pathology, and microbiology by small faculties of mostly physician educators and scientists, although, to be sure, a few prominent PhD investigators were involved in the enterprise. A similar model was in place in Europe, where most medical schools did not offer PhD training and most medical school researchers, including the likes of Krebs and Ehrlich, were physicians. In many European countries, medical school professors performing biomedical research had significantly greater societal stature, and in many cases earned a higher income, than practicing clinicians.

During this period academic physicians often saw patients and conducted research simultaneously—usually in modest laboratories in the
hospital or even in their offices. Laboratories existed without the structure of academic departments, and research, though small in scale, was
highly collaborative, often involving students and clinically undifferen-
tiated postgraduate trainees. A good example of the times is Frederick
Banting (Banting 1965), who, though originally trained as an orthopedic
surgeon, became interested in diabetes and moved from London, Ontario,
to Toronto to work with the physician-scientist John Macleod, recently recruited from Cleveland to the university to be professor of physiology.
With critical help from a PhD student, Charles Best, they utilized a dog
model of diabetes and eventually isolated and characterized insulin, an
accomplishment for which Banting and Macleod shared a Nobel Prize. In
Boston, the Thorndike Laboratory in the old Boston City Hospital became
an incubator for physiological approaches to anemia (Elrod and Karnad
2003). There the physicians George Minot and George Murphy built on
the recent discoveries of another physician, George Whipple, to develop
a cure for pernicious anemia, for which they shared a Nobel Prize. Later
at the Thorndike Lab their trainee William Castle ingeniously discovered
Intrinsic Factor as the critical gastric protein required for vitamin B12
absorption.

Although human physiology and biomedical research during this early
era were largely the purview of physician-scientists, the seeds were planted
to grow the new medical research fields of biochemistry, molecular biology, genetics, and cell and developmental biology. Perhaps the first examples of modern "translational" research came in these early days when
basic tools and principles of the physical sciences, such as chromatogra-
phy, spectroscopy, centrifugation, crystallography, and X-ray diffraction
analysis, were applied to biology. This led to the emergence of techniques
to image cells in fine detail and to purify and analyze proteins and other
macromolecules. Much of this work was done in university laboratories
by PhD scientists. Men such as J. D. Bernal, Max Perutz, John Kendrew,
and Frederick Sanger at Cambridge and Linus Pauling at Cal Tech, and
women such as Rosalind Franklin at King's College, London, were PhD
scientists trained in chemistry and physics. Nonetheless, they had enormous impact on the future of biomedicine by showing how physical techniques could be used to understand protein (and later DNA) structure
and, significantly, how structure could be used to understand function
(Ferry 2007). It has been reported that Pauling's decision to study hemoglobin from patients with sickle cell disease was suggested by William
Castle on a long train ride from Boston to Denver (Bunn 2007). Castle had

noted that when red cells from these patients sickled, they changed shape and showed birefringence in polarized light. Theorizing that a specific molecular realignment or reorientation must be occurring, he urged Pauling to pursue this topic. A year or two later Pauling demonstrated that the single amino acid substitution in the hemoglobin molecule responsible for sickle cell disease induced dramatic oxygen tension–dependent changes in the physicochemical properties of the molecule, hence describing what he termed the first "molecular" disease (Pauling et al. 1949).

Along with physiology, the other dominant field of medical research in this era was focused on understanding the microbiological basis of infectious diseases, then the most pressing public health problem worldwide. Here we find many examples of physicians who cared for patients who also applied their intellectual skills to the bench. Oswald Avery, for example, was a clinician interested in the bacteriology of pneumonia. After getting his start at the Hoagland Laboratory in Brooklyn, he moved to the Rockefeller Institute in New York (now Rockefeller University), where his association with two other prominent physician-scientists, Maclyn McCarty and Colin Macleod, and their studies of the pneumococcus bacterium led to the identification of DNA as the carrier of genetic information. Similarly, Renato Dulbeco and Salvatore Luria, two Nobel Prize–winning physician-scientists who were initially trained in Turin, made groundbreaking discoveries on the nature of genetic mutations using bacteriophage. The work of these early investigators, placed in the context of the relatively recent "rediscovery" of Mendelian genetics and the development by PhD scientists, including Thomas Hunt Morgan, of simple model systems such as drosophila (fruit flies) to use as genetic tools, laid the groundwork for the development of modern genetics. This field, of course, soon exploded with the discovery of the structure of DNA by Watson and Crick. The fact that Luria served as James Watson's PhD thesis adviser in genetics at Indiana University provides an outstanding example of the importance of fostering interactions between MD scientists and PhD scientists.

Although interactions among physicians and PhD scientists were well documented and often extremely fruitful during this early era of biomedical research, most medical research was performed by physicians with a consuming interest in the critical diseases of the era. These physicians were well trained in the preclinical sciences of physiology and microbiology, and were relatively unencumbered by regulatory and funding burdens or other academic responsibilities. The technologic gap between physician and PhD investigators was small. For physician-scientists it was easily solved by short visits to laboratories of other scientists to learn new techniques as they evolved or by inviting other scientists into their laboratories for brief visits. The biomedical research literature was much more limited than today, and it was not unusual for researchers to read from cover to cover every issue of, for example, the *Journal of Biological Chemistry* as soon as it arrived. For PhD scientists who wished to learn more of the medical relevance of their research, opportunities to engage physician-scientists in leisurely conversations abounded at research symposia, academic events, and scientific society meetings. Clinical medicine in that era was relatively crude, so basic discoveries could be translated to the clinic fairly quickly, often with dramatic results. In 1921, when Banting began his work on diabetes, the average life expectancy of a child newly diagnosed with Type 1 diabetes was less than twelve months. Shortly after his team first isolated insulin, in January 1922, they treated their first patient: the desperately ill fourteen-year-old Leonard Thompson, who ultimately went on to live another thirteen years (Banting 1965). By the end of that year insulin was being produced commercially and was used widely. Similarly, it did not take a cadre of well-trained clinical trialists to bring antibiotic therapy forward for bacterial pneumonia, or B12 therapy for pernicious anemia. These examples are not meant to imply, however, that no translational gap existed. Despite Pauling's success in "solving" sickle cell disease at the molecular and thermodynamic level in the 1940s, we still do not have a specific effective therapy today.

Modern History of MD-PhD Interactions

The advances in biomedical research during the first half of the twentieth century created enormous opportunities. After the Second World War, when resources (especially in the United States) became available to expand the community of biomedical scientists and support science on a national level, there was a tremendously receptive substrate available to receive the largess and reap the rewards. An unintended consequence, however, was the independent growth trajectories of basic and clinical departments at academic medical centers, which contributed to a general loss of connection between clinical and basic investigators. To a large extent this can be traced to the exponential growth of the NIH under what became known as the "Shannon Doctrine" (Shannon 1987; Wyngaarden 1987; Eichna 1972). James Shannon was one of the earliest MD-PhD investigators. He had obtained his PhD in physiology at New York University in 1935 after completing medical school there in 1929 and then residency training at Bellevue Hospital. In a short period of time he made several major contributions to the field of renal physiology before taking a detour during World War II to study antimalarial therapies at Goldwater

Hospital in New York. After the war he spent a few years in the pharmaceutical industry researching antibiotics and then worked in an administrative position at the NIH National Heart Institute, the forerunner of what is now the National Heart, Lung and Blood Institute.

Shannon—a persuasive spokesman and leader—was an extraordinary advocate for science in Congress, the executive branch, and the halls of academic medicine. In 1955 he was appointed director of the NIH, where, over his thirteen-year tenure, he oversaw its expansion from an agency with a $180 million annual budget to one with $1.2 billion to spend in his last year. With this almost sevenfold budgetary expansion, American biomedical science became an "enterprise" rather than a cottage industry. Academic medical centers largely superseded universities and community hospitals as sites for training and research.

Shannon's advocacy was based on a few simple guiding principles that set the stage for the direction of growth of the medical research enterprise. He emphatically believed that diseases could be cured only through fundamental biological understanding of their root causes. He also insisted that government-sponsored research should be broad in scope and ongoing in nature, and that the individual scientist was the driving force for innovation. With the universal acceptance of these principles, academic medical centers throughout the country developed their "preclinical" operations at a rapid pace. They created and enlarged basic science departments to support a rapidly growing cadre of NIH R01-funded laboratory investigators who were performing basic biologic research and mechanistic studies on human disease. Grant-derived faculty salary support and indirect cost recovery allowed significant expansion of research departments without causing a drain on the department's internal funds. Along with this growth of preclinical departments was a concomitant increase in the clinical departments that paralleled the emergence of multiple new specialties. Each department had its own administrative structure and residency training program and often its own NIH-funded laboratory research program.

By the late 1960s, when Shannon stepped down from the NIH, biomedical science had become "big business." In the decades that followed, NIH budgets continued their remarkable rise, and academic medical centers built more and more research buildings, often physically disconnected from the practicing physicians and hospitals. Medical center directors and deans grew dependent on the indirect cost recovery from the NIH generated by their "individual innovators"—the R01-funded basic scientists. Physician-investigators were increasingly drawn to the excitement of laboratory-based research. Many became enamored with the scientific revolution precipitated by the rapid developments in molecular biology and the resultant new tools to study the basic pathophysiology of human disease. A new culture emerged of the academic physician-scientist who was a laboratory researcher and teacher, but often quite removed from the day-to-day clinical world (Goldstein and Brown 1997).

Few, however, would argue with the phenomenal successes that came from investing in basic and disease-oriented research. The model of using disease to learn about basic biology has been repeatedly validated, and who better to study diseases than physicians? It was, after all, clinically trained investigators, such as Nobel laureates Michael Brown and Joseph Goldstein, who unraveled the mysteries of receptor-mediated endocytosis by studying cells from their patients with familial hypercholesterolemia. It was Stanley Korsmeyer who identified the mitochondrial pathway of apoptosis by studying his patients with follicular lymphoma. These discoveries and contributions were enormously enriched by the collaborative relationship of these investigators with PhD scientists from the fields of classical cell biology, biochemistry, genetics, and model organism developmental biology. Of course such major discoveries were not limited to physician-scientists with direct patient contact. PhD scientists made many discoveries with profound and immediate relationships to clinical medicine. Most of these PhDs were untrained in clinical work, but they created affiliations with clinicians who had access to patients and patient-derived materials. Louis Kunkel's discovery of the role of the muscle protein dystrophin, and Mary Claire King's discovery of the tumor-suppressor gene BRCA-1, came from their success in establishing partnerships with the physicians who cared for patients afflicted with muscular dystrophy or breast cancer (Davies and White 1995).

Certain areas of medical research have remained extremely collaborative and multidisciplinary in nature, perhaps the best example, as noted earlier, being human disease genetics. Our own research areas, vascular biology and thrombosis, are also marked by a continuing tradition of cross-disciplinary interactions. In 1945 at the Cleveland Clinic, Irvine Page, MD, the discoverer of serotonin, assembled a multidisciplinary team of physiologists, chemists, physicists, and clinicians to focus on hypertension (Clough 2004). The team's efforts led to the discovery and synthesis of angiotensin and many other major contributions to defining the renin-angiotensin system. Continued multidisciplinary efforts at the national level have been fostered in the modern era by NIH support for multi-investigator team research in the form of so-called Center Grants and Program Project Grants. Organizations such as the American Heart Association, North American Vascular Biology Organization, American

Society of Investigative Pathology, and American Society of Hematology (ASH) have also promoted a tradition of inclusiveness. This tradition includes joint participation in study sections, editorial boards, and meeting program planning, and support of both MD and PhD training and career development. It is worth noting that the incoming president of ASH as of this writing was Hal Broxmeyer, a PhD scientist who has made groundbreaking translational discoveries related to hematopoietic stem cells. That an organization of nearly fourteen thousand members, of whom the vast majority are physicians, would elect a basic scientist as president must reflect a broad acceptance within the medical community of the value of PhD-MD collaborations.

Despite these dramatic collaborative success stories, the loss of consistent, widespread interactions between basic and clinical investigators has persisted, and has probably contributed to the translational research gap. Many explanations have been put forward to explain the continued loss of interactions (Wyngaarden 1979; Goldstein and Brown 1997; Kelley and Randolph 1994). One points to the physical and administrative barriers that have been created in academia which separate departments and programs from one another. The evolution of many medical school curricula to nondepartmental-based models that have transferred many teaching responsibilities (and hence contacts with medical students and physician educators) out of the realm of the basic science departments also feeds the problem. Another exacerbating factor is the narrow focus of many basic scientists on R01-fundable research projects motivated by highly competitive NIH paylines.

Contributing to the disconnect between PhD and physician investigators is the growing knowledge gap between the clinician or clinical researcher and the laboratory-based researcher. This gap exists on both sides of the aisle. The tools and technologies of clinical and population-based research have developed at a rapid pace as these scientific disciplines have matured. Knowledge of the complex statistical and informatics technologies required for these disciplines is not part of most PhD training programs, nor is instruction in the complex regulatory requirements for human subjects research. Furthermore, the predominant place of molecular biology, cell biology, and genetics in most PhD training programs has displaced whole organismal physiology from most curricula. Most PhD scientists have little understanding of the "whole animal" implications of a molecular or genetic discovery.

On the other side, the preclinical component of the medical school curriculum in most schools has evolved to include more clinical experiences during the first two years (at the expense of basic science time). This leaves little or no time for instruction in the complex cross-disciplinary scientific topics such as genomics, proteomics, bioinformatics, structural biology, and imaging that are driving modern science. In the end, physicians are not prepared to understand the research of most PhD scientists, and PhD scientists are not prepared to understand the research of the clinical, patient-oriented investigators.

Moving Forward into the Twenty-first Century

Academic and government leaders now recognize that overcoming the translational research gap is a high priority as biomedical science moves forward. They also understand that building bridges between the basic science and clinical science research communities is likely to be a key step in successful and rapid translation. It has become important therefore to identify the roadblocks to bridge building and to develop novel strategies to overcome them. These can be divided conceptually into two categories: those that relate to new training strategies for MD and/or PhD scientists, and those that relate to reengineering structures within academic medical centers to foster interactions between clinical and basic researchers.

Training Strategies for Physicians to Enhance Interactions with Basic Scientists

Perhaps the earliest attempt to integrate significant research training into the medical school years dates to 1964, with the development of the NIH-funded Medical Scientist Training Program (MSTP) to support combined MD-PhD training for a highly select group of entering medical students. The rationale for the program was that dual training in both medicine and rigorous biomedical science would yield a cohort of physician-scientists capable of moving easily between the clinical and basic research arenas. The program has grown significantly in scale and scope since its inception, with the large majority of medical schools now offering the dual degree option. Since the NIH program supports tuition and provides cost-of-living stipends, a major advantage to these students is the ability to graduate from medical school largely unencumbered by debt, hence able to choose a career pathway that involves a significant delay in time before realizing their full economic earning potential.

In light of many years' experience with the MD-PhD concept (Lin 1999), there is agreement that the program has been successful in creating a cadre of exceptionally successful physician-scientists who are mainly focused on disease-relevant basic laboratory research. As detailed in chapter 2 by Timothy Ley, MD-PhD investigators compete better than

MD-only or PhD-only investigators for NIH R01 grants. MD-PhDs are also well represented in academic faculties, in academic and industry leadership, and in the honorific research societies, such as the American Society for Clinical Investigation, Institute of Medicine, and National Academy of Sciences. Little evidence exists, however, to support the hypothesis that this group has significantly addressed the gap in patient-oriented clinical and translational research. This probably reflects a selection bias in that most schools choose their MD-PhD students on the basis of interest, aptitude, and previous experience with basic biological science. Also, even in the absence of debt, the lengthy process required for "full" training in both medicine and research is problematic. Moving through medical school to graduate coursework with a research thesis, then to postgraduate clinical training (which averages six years for most specialties), and finally to additional postgraduate research training to catch up after the clinical training hiatus is off-putting to most graduates who may have begun the program with the goal of becoming a clinical investigator (Haspel 2006).

Recognizing that the dual MD-PhD programs have not resulted in significantly changing the national balance between basic and translational researchers, the academic and funding communities have explored other options. To a large extent these have involved programs to provide research training to physicians, but at less depth and in less time than the MSTP and often integrated into the standard medical or graduate medical education programs. The Harvard-MIT Health Sciences and Technology (HST) Program (Gray and Bonventre 2002), begun in 1970, is a consortium involving the two universities and the Harvard teaching hospitals that offers a broad range of educational activities, including an academic track within the Harvard Medical School MD program. It includes a research curriculum and thesis experience. Sixty percent of the students in this track do not pursue PhD degrees, but many spend an extra year or two in medical school. The HST programs also include postgraduate research training for physicians in clinical research and in focused biomedical and bioengineering science areas, including imaging, informatics, and regenerative medicine.

Other programs that embed research training into the medical school education experience include Duke University School of Medicine and the Cleveland Clinic Lerner College of Medicine of Case Western Reserve University, established in 2004. The former compresses the standard two-year medical school preclinical curriculum to accommodate a mandatory year of research. The latter is an innovative five-year program that includes a formal curriculum in both clinical and laboratory research as well as a mandatory one-year research experience with thesis. In addition to these innovative approaches, the Howard Hughes Medical Institute, Sarnoff Foundation, and other organizations provide financial support to a limited number of medical students to take a year-long hiatus from medical school to pursue supervised research. The net result of all these initiatives and programs is that a substantially larger number of medical students graduate each year with significant research experience than was the case twenty or so years ago. These students often work in laboratories directed by PhD scientists and often side by side with PhD students and postdoctoral fellows.

While these programs are all built on lofty goals and the sound principle that early research exposure is a critical predictive event in "capturing" students into research careers, most of these programs segregate the research experience as extracurricular and "independent." While these efforts are likely to have a positive impact on the size of the clinical/translational research community, it remains unclear what their true "yield" will be. How many of these students will ultimately pursue clinical or translational research as part of their careers?

Programs like those at the Cleveland Clinic and the Harvard-MIT HST that include formal exposure to certain key elements of successful translational research (e.g., advanced basic science and clinical research methodologies courses, and experience with the assembly, operations, and added value of multidisciplinary research teams that include both MD and PhD investigators) are more directly addressing the translational research gap. We hope that they will develop outcomes data validating their approach.

At the graduate medical education (GME) level numerous approaches have been taken to increase the pool of clinical and translational researchers, including the embedding of formal graduate coursework toward MS and PhD degrees into clinical training programs. These have been particularly successful in health services and clinical epidemiology research but largely unproved in the realm of clinical/translational research.

Graduate schools in association with clinical departments have developed several particularly innovative programs. For example, the STAR program at the David Geffen School of Medicine at UCLA offers the opportunity to combine clinical residency or fellowship training with advanced research training. Trainees can emerge with both clinical board eligibility and either a PhD in a basic science or health services field or an MS degree in clinical research. The research portion of the program is usually three to four years in duration, but salary support commensurate with clinical training level and tuition costs is provided throughout the training period. Yale also provides formal training in clinical investigation to physicians in clinical departments. It offers them an opportunity to earn a PhD degree in investigative medicine in a timeframe "not substantially different from that required for research training in most medical subspecialties," as its website states. The NIH has provided competitive funding to institutions for postgraduate research curriculum development and support through its K30 and K12 programs. (Both are mentored research training grants, with the former dedicated specifically to clinical research.) These have been effective at helping program directors incorporate formal instruction in clinical trial design, biostatistics, research ethics, and clinical epidemiology into clinical training. For the most part, however, they have not addressed training in translational research or in working within multidisciplinary teams that include both MD and PhD investigators.

A major obstacle to the success of all of these GME-based programs is the failure of the major credentialing organizations, such as the American Specialty Boards and the Accreditation Council for Graduate Medical Education (ACGME), to align clinical training objectives with research training objectives. Thus for an individual trainee or program director it becomes very difficult to ensure that all of the requirements for board certification are satisfied without significantly extending the training period. Extension of training raises difficult financial concerns for programs, since clinical department budgets are under extreme stress, and hospitals are unlikely to provide support for non-GME-required activities. This puts the trainee in the difficult position of trying to find extramural support and/or clinical "moonlighting" opportunities to make ends meet while further extending the time before initiating an academic faculty appointment (and commensurate salary). Since many trainees at this point in their career are also starting families, any extension of training becomes a major disincentive.

Given the national "crisis" in translational research and the imperative to increase the number and improve the quality of translational researchers, it is not unreasonable for the boards, the ACGME, professional specialty societies, and training program directors to become active partners in the solution. It is critical that these groups recognize that clinical careers are becoming increasingly subspecialized and that it is unreasonable to expect all specialty graduates to be experts in all aspects of a complex field. It is also essential that they validate the importance of clinical and translational research in all fields by redesigning specialty training requirements to allow an expanded research experience without lengthening the entire training process.

Training Strategies for PhD Scientists to Enhance
Interactions with Clinicians

The inherent complexity and excitement of both modern biomedical science and modern clinical medicine make it extremely unlikely that medical school curricula will ever be able to provide students with sufficient scientific background to become effective translational researchers without significant expansion of what is already an extremely long training period. Thus, despite the valiant efforts described earlier, the solution to the translational research gap cannot rely solely on better training of physician-scientists in the tools and techniques of translational research. A logical source of new intellectual capital for this enterprise is the pool of biomedical scientists trained in PhD programs. Most graduate students pursuing biomedical research PhDs in the United States are enrolled in programs located within or affiliated with medical schools. The vast majority of these students indicate that their choice was based on a desire to pursue "medically relevant" research (Gray and Bonventre 2007). They are therefore a receptive cohort for career development in translational research.

Until the 1970s the curriculum for most students in biomedical PhD programs in American medical schools began with the traditional first-year preclinical medical school courses (including anatomy and physiology), which they usually took along with the medical students, but with the addition of extra sessions for more in-depth study. With the emergence of the "molecular era," however, this translational model was uniformly dropped. Most current PhD programs are locked into a model wherein students complete a separate, relatively standard core curriculum focused on intensive exposure to molecular biology, biochemistry, genetics, and cell biology, with pharmacology, immunology, or neuroscience added on for some.

Students then enter a research laboratory, where they complete a highly focused "mechanistic" research thesis project under the direction of a single mentor. Most of these graduate students have little or no interaction with physicians or medical students and little or no experience working as part of a multidisciplinary team. Thus for a PhD student in the modern era to become an effective translational researcher, knowledge gaps in organismal and population biology, pathophysiologic and pharmacologic principles, and regulatory aspects of human subjects research must be addressed. Furthermore, students must learn how to communicate with physicians and physician-scientists to participate effectively as members of multidisciplinary teams.

Several attempts have been made to create training pathways for PhD students that address some of these needs. Perhaps the most mature of these are the ones based in bioengineering departments at such institutions as Johns Hopkins, Harvard-MIT (HST), and the University of California. The HST Medical Engineering and Medical Physics PhD program (Gray and Bonventre 2007), established in the late 1970s, includes coursework in either systems physiology or cell and molecular biology taken side by side with Harvard medical students and MD-PhD students. This is then followed by an intensive clinical experience with hands-on patient contact.

This program has had documented success in graduating academically oriented biomedical engineers, many of whom are publishing in top-tier medical research journals, and many whose primary faculty appointments are in clinical departments. The relationship of translational and team-oriented research to the applied science of engineering is of course much more obvious than to molecular and cellular biology. Nevertheless, in parallel to the HST model, several other graduate schools began experimenting with clinical experiences for PhD students in the 1980s. The program developed at Tufts University by Irwin Arias is well documented (Arias 1989). In this program students take a one-semester pathobiology course that includes patient interactions, exposure to major diagnostic and therapeutic facilities, and instruction and readings in basic pathophysiologic principles.

Motivated by the apparent successes of the HST and Tufts programs, the Lucille P. Markey Charitable Trust, which existed as a limited-term philanthropic fund between 1983 and 1998, awarded grants intended to catalyze new ways to train PhD students in translational research. In addition to HST and Tufts, several additional programs were funded, including one at Washington University and one at Cornell Medical College (Bond et al. 2004). Unfortunately, since the new curricula and clinical exposure programs at most of the schools were funded entirely by the grant, most had no resources to sustain the programs when the trust ceased operations. Sadly, most of the programs no longer exist. Equally unfortunate, limited outcomes data are available though the program ran for more than ten years, and a significant amount of money was spent.

Given the obvious national need, the limited but generally positive outcomes data, and the anecdotal sense from the Markey program directors that these programs tended to attract outstanding graduate students, interest in adding similar clinical curricula to traditional graduate programs has persisted. In 2007 the Cleveland Clinic, through its academic affiliate Case Western Reserve University School of Medicine, began offering a PhD program in molecular medicine. Its goal was to train PhD scientists who were comfortable with and knowledgeable in the practice of multi-disciplinary clinical and translational research. The program is designed to fill the knowledge gaps outlined previously by providing an integrated fourteen-month core curriculum that begins with an introduction to mammalian systems physiology linked to clinical cases as examples. Students then follow a curriculum that links biochemistry, metabolism, cell and molecular biology, genetics, and immunology/host defense with clinical diseases as examples.

A unique component of the core course is an intensive ten-week block called "Clinical and Translational Research for the Laboratory Scientist," in which the students are exposed to core principles of human subjects research, including subject consent and recruitment, biomarker development, clinical informatics, bioethics, regulatory principles, translational research methods, commercialization and technology transfer, and basic clinical epidemiology and biostatistics. Beginning with their second year of graduate school, when they choose a thesis research mentor and laboratory project, they are assigned a clinical co–thesis mentor who will work with them throughout the remainder of their graduate experience. The two mentors together design a longitudinal clinical experience for the student that is complementary to his or her laboratory research. The experience includes participation in a multidisciplinary clinical and clinical research conference, as well as direct interaction with clinicians in various settings, including diagnostic and therapeutic. Goals of the program include exposure of the students to the "face" of human disease and to the obstacles to effective clinical research. This helps them understand how clinicians determine research priorities, as well as learn how to engage a multi-disciplinary team that includes physicians. The program is supported by one of a small number of grants from the Howard Hughes Medical Institute (HHMI) as part of its "Med to Grad" initiative. It is intended to support various approaches to injecting medicine into PhD training programs in biomedicine and engineering.

Another PhD program in "Translational Research and Molecular Medicine" has been launched at Baylor College of Medicine in Houston. Also funded by the HHMI initiative, the program reported that interactions between "clinical mentor" and "basic mentor" during the first three years of the program had already resulted in more than a dozen new translational collaborations. Since program assessment is built into the HHMI grant programs, important data should become available that other funding agencies and graduate programs can use to design and support programs with similar goals.

Reengineering Academic Structures to Enhance Interactions

The administrative structures within most academic medical centers were well designed to support the rapid growth in basic research and clinical medicine during the latter half of the last century. Unfortunately, the centrifugal forces generated by rapid expansion led to compartmentalization of research and training within departments and divisions and separation and physical isolation of basic science departments from clinical activities. Furthermore, promotion and tenure committees became driven by the metrics that generated growth and are the easiest to quantify: the individual R01 grant and first or last author publications in the "high-impact" journals. Lost in this evolution was the understanding or appreciation of accomplishments within multidisciplinary collaborative groups. Thus architecture, culture, and governance developed in ways that create significant barriers to translational research and to productive interactions between PhD and MD investigators.

As medical centers mature and the NIH continues to pump more financial resources into translational and multidisciplinary research, we are beginning to see significant reengineering of academic structures. Many academic medical centers are changing their patient care models from the traditional departmental basis to the "service line" model, in which physicians from multiple specialties are clustered to provide efficient and multidisciplinary care. In these models the service line director has administrative and leadership responsibilities that cross traditional academic boundaries. The earliest examples are the cancer centers that are now ubiquitous at academic and community medical centers. Many institutions are developing similar approaches to cardiovascular, neurological, musculoskeletal, metabolic, and other diseases. Cleveland Clinic has gone as far as eliminating its old departmental structure and substituting an "institute" model in which all clinical departments and divisions have been re-clustered on the basis of this principle.

While the service line models have greatly facilitated clinical research, the next major challenge is to incorporate disease-oriented basic laboratory research into the teams. With significant financial motivation coming from the NIH, this is beginning to occur. The National Cancer Institute (NCI), through its Comprehensive Cancer Center designation, was a driving force in the initial development of academic cancer centers. Renewal of these large infrastructure grants requires demonstration of significant interaction between laboratory researchers and clinical researchers and significant central institutional support for these activities. It has become common for PhD cancer biologists to meet frequently with clinical oncologists in disease-specific multidisciplinary conferences and for both groups to participate jointly in research projects. These interactions are producing better-organized strategies for tumor biobanking, clinical phenotyping, DNA profiling, and other broad-based approaches to facilitate translational research. As other NIH institutes begin to encourage translational research through their extramural centers and programs, there is likely to be a similar positive effect.

An interesting model is Cleveland Clinic, where the basic science departments under the umbrella of a research institute have long been organized around disease-oriented research rather than classical academic disciplines. The institute is considered a "matrix" organization, and the ten individual departments and approximately 150 independent principal investigators are charged with building bridges to the clinical institutes to facilitate research and educational cooperation. A motivating factor is that the annual performance review of all departments and individuals includes an assessment of these cooperative activities.

Perhaps the biggest change agent in facilitating these reengineering efforts is the NIH, through its Clinical Translational Science Award (CTSA) program (Butler 2008). The national network of CTSAs supported by $500 million in annual NIH funding is envisioned as a driving force to support and sustain clinical and translational research. In so doing, it is fostering change in local cultures to provide an "academic home" for clinical and translational investigators. CTSA-funded centers are empowered to encourage multidisciplinary research involving both PhD and MD scientists by providing pilot project funding and cross-training opportunities. Significantly, infrastructures are being built to enable PhD investigators to communicate with clinicians, access clinical information and samples, and develop translational strategies for basic discoveries. At the same time, infrastructures are being built to enable MD investigators to communicate with basic scientists and access complex laboratory technologies to provide translational support for clinical investigation. It is hoped that institutions will leverage CTSA resources to expand translational research across all disciplines and encourage formation of multidisciplinary research teams that include MDs and PhDs, nurses, pharmacists, engineers, and other professionals broadly involved in the medical research enterprise.

Summary

The relationship between PhD scientists and physicians has undergone substantial evolution during the one hundred–year period since the Flexner

Report. Although there has never been uniformity across academic institutions or scientific fields, a general drifting apart of the two groups occurred during the latter part of the twentieth century as medical centers became larger and basic science departments became less involved with medical student education and less connected to clinical departments. With the realization that the gap between basic discovery and clinical implementation was reaching a crisis, and that at least part of the solution to this problem lay in providing encouragement and incentive for research collaborations across multiple fields of study, steps are being taken nationally to facilitate interactions between physicians and basic scientists. Individual institutions are piloting various models of new training paradigms at the pre- and postgraduate levels. They are also experimenting with new cross-disciplinary care delivery and research models. The invisible hand of the NIH and other large funding agencies will no doubt continue to drive these changes, and the entrepreneurial spirit of American medicine and academia is likely to continue to produce innovative solutions. In the end, the more that physicians and PhD scientists share ideas and work together, the greater will be the acceleration in translational discoveries.

10

Mentoring Physician-Scientists

REPAIRING THE LEAKY PIPELINE

Kenneth Kaushansky, MD

Physician-scientists are individuals with medical training who spend most or all of their time performing disease-oriented or patient-oriented research. Physician-scientists are critical members of the medical research community, as the scientific questions they ask derive from taking care of patients. While the pathway to becoming a physician-scientist can be varied, there are two basic models. One is represented by the MD-PhD who entered a combined degree program after graduation from college and has had a clear path toward a career in biomedical science. The alternate pathway, characterized by many as the "late bloomer," comprises approximately two-thirds to three-quarters of all physician-scientists. These physicians have first completed their clinical training and only then embarked on a serious pursuit of biomedical science. Mentoring of each of these types of individuals varies mainly on the basis of the need to provide additional scientific training. The two groups, however, also confront many similar issues that stem from the long-term commitment physician-scientists make as they develop their skills in both medicine and science. This dual mastery, or bilingualism as I refer to it, is critical, since the full-time clinician does not and should not accept suboptimal patient care from the physician-scientist; nor does the PhD scientist hold the physician-scientist to a lesser standard of excellence than that used to judge his or her peers who are full-time researchers. Hence, mentoring becomes a necessity, not a luxury.

The Leaky Pipeline: Physician-Scientists Are Falling Behind

Recent statistics reveal very slow growth of medical scientist training programs (MD-PhD or MSTP) programs and an overall loss of well-trained physician-scientists, including MD-PhDs, to clinical practice (Varki and Rosenberg 2002). This relative reduction is due to a myriad of conditions, discussed at length in other chapters of this volume. For the purposes of this discussion, important factors that contribute include the increased time necessary for completion of clinical training; a perceived inadequacy of research training for MDs; economic disincentives including low stipends, increasing debt burden, and income disparities between physicians in private practice and academia; the instability of NIH-supported research careers; the explosive growth of managed care; and increasing demand for physicians to see more patients coupled with declining departmental revenues that can be used to support research through intramural sources.

Collectively these factors have resulted in a major change in academic medical centers, one that is toxic to spawning young investigators. Instead of hearing about the remarkable scientific opportunities that lie ahead, medical students hear about how difficult it is to get research funds. Instead of being told what a wonderful career successful investigators enjoy, residents are told how little time investigators have for research. Instead of witnessing their mentors practicing an academic lifestyle devoted to teaching and discovering, fellows see faculty harried and harassed by the heavy institutional pressure of the financial "bottom line." Should it surprise us that students are not flocking to emulate their physician-scientist teachers? It is the underlying hypothesis of this chapter that enhancements in mentoring will increase the rate at which bright and energetic young people enter the pool of nascent physician-scientists and reduce the loss of talented, well-trained physician-scientists into clinical careers. And while great mentoring is not a certain cure for the leaky physician-scientist career pipeline, poor mentoring is guaranteed to turn any leaks into a torrent. Moreover, academic leaders must focus on collective mentoring. Rather than bemoan our fate in discouraging editorials, I would suggest we embrace the scientific accomplishments of our times and make certain we do not convey an attitude that the cup is half empty.

Mentor: The Myth and the Modern

Classical Greek mythology tells us that, upon embarking on the his travels made famous by Homer, Odysseus chose Mentor to watch over his son

Telemachos. Athena, the Greek goddess of wisdom, was said to occupy
Mentor's body to impart knowledge to Telemachos. In more contemporary times, the term *mentor* has been used synonymously with *adviser,
teacher, coach, tutor,* and *advocate.*

The sociologist Morris Zelditch summarized a mentor's multiple roles:
"Mentors are advisors, people with career experience willing to share
their knowledge; supporters, people who give emotional and moral encouragement; tutors, people who give specific feedback on one's performance; masters, in the sense of employers to whom one is apprenticed;
sponsors, sources of information about and aid in obtaining opportunities;
models, of identity, of the kind of person one should be to be an academic"
(Council of Graduate Schools 1995). The ideal mentor is a good listener;
is aware of the amount of attention needed by different learners, including those who do not ask for help; and is available to provide it. The ideal
mentor is also a great problem solver, but one who does not spoon-feed
his or her protégé. And an effective mentor acknowledges that a single
individual cannot know everything a given student might need in order to
succeed. For example, a survey of over 1,400 faculty members at the University of Pennsylvania School of Medicine found that the more facets of
mentoring provided to a junior faculty mentor, the more favorable his or
her job satisfaction rating and the less likelihood of his or her leaving the
institution. This study also found that the more mentors a junior faculty
member identified, the greater the number of types of mentoring that was
provided (Wasserstein, Quistberg, and Shea 2007).

Classic Mentoring: The Experienced Mentor
and the Physician-Scientist Trainee

A mentor may be defined as an active partner in an ongoing relationship
who helps a learner maximize potential and reach personal and professional goals. Research in law, business, and nursing has shown that mentoring leads to higher levels of career satisfaction and a higher rate of
promotion, with a greater effect if it begins early in a person's career (Ramanan et al. 2002). From the outset one must admit that there are precious
few rigorous data supporting a role for mentoring in the successful development of physician-scientists. One literature search (Sambunjak, Straus,
and Marusi 2006) identified 3,640 citations on mentoring in academic
medicine; of these, only forty-two articles describing thirty-nine studies
were deemed appropriate for inclusion in the review.

Unfortunately, while mentoring is perceived as an important part of
academic medicine, the evidence to support this perception is not strong.

For example, a poll of approximately three thousand full-time U.S. medical school faculty members boasted a 60 percent response rate that was roughly equally distributed between those with and without mentors. Compared to those without, junior faculty with mentors published an equal number of peer-reviewed papers, were more likely to obtain a research grant, and had higher levels of career satisfaction (Palepu et al. 1998). I do not believe that any physician-scientist would consider this study a rigorous examination of the success of mentoring. Altogether, the best that can be said of an objective look at the medical literature reflecting various survey strategies is that fellows and junior faculty members with mentors enjoy greater career satisfaction than those without. They also *perceive* themselves to have higher academic performance (presentation and grant writing skills and research productivity). Nevertheless, while as a biomedical scientist and clinician I pride myself on evaluating and making decisions on only the most rigorous of data, I will push on with this chapter, knowing that it is not overwhelmingly evidence based.

Examples of Key Contributions of Physician-Scientists and Their Mentors

Since the inception of the Nobel Prize in 1901, 101 of 172 laureates in medicine and physiology held MD degrees (Archer 2007). The achievements of Nobel laureates generally better reflect persistence than prescience. While the following stories are anecdotal, they are nevertheless important and highly visible illustrations.

Alfred Nobel studied with Jules Pelouze, inventor of guncotton, working beside Ascanio Sobero, inventor of nitroglycerin. Prompted by his brother Emil's death, the result of a nitroglycerin explosion, Alfred invented dynamite, a stabilized form of nitroglycerin. In Nobel's lifetime, physicians learned the therapeutic value of nitroglycerin for angina pectoris. Paradoxically, Nobel refused treatment with nitroglycerin for his chest pain, remarking, "Isn't it the irony of fate that I have been prescribed nitroglycerin, to be taken internally!"

Willem Einthoven won the Nobel Prize in 1924 for his development of the clinical electrocardiogram in 1903. Einthoven's contributions to the emerging field included incorporating advances in electromagnetism, recording technology, optics, and quartz chemistry to create a recording system that produced traces of excellent quality. Einthoven acknowledged that his work was built on that of others, including Thomas Lewis, the father of clinical electrocardiography, who was overlooked for the prize, stating, "The general interest in ECG would certainly not have risen so high without his [Lewis's] work." The realization that making major incremental discoveries is highly meritorious should encourage young physician-scientists. Frans Cornelis Donders pointed Einthoven toward the study of cardiac electrical activity, and also assisted him in becoming professor of physiology at the University of Leiden. This illustrates two of the key roles played by mentors: helping to establish the "big question" and providing opportunities to explore.

Peter Agre won the 2003 Nobel Prize in chemistry for his discovery of aquaporins, or water channels. A product of the turbulent 1960s, Agre completed his chemistry degree and entered Johns Hopkins School of Medicine. Medicine appealed to Agre as a way of addressing global health issues. Yet during a research internship working on cholera toxin with pharmacologist Pedro Cuatrecasas, Agre was transformed. He later explained the experience: "You know that scene in *The Wizard of Oz* where Dorothy wakes up and suddenly everything is in color? That's what it was like for me in Pedro's lab." Following his residency in internal medicine and a fellowship in hematology-oncology at the University of North Carolina, Agre again took to the laboratory. He worked with Vann Bennett, then at Burroughs Wellcome, who kindled his interest in red blood cell proteins. Of the first of the aquaporins to be purified, Agre noted: "When we first identified this protein, ironically we thought it was a contaminant. A wiser scientist might have said, 'Well, just disregard the dirt and concentrate on the important stuff.' But we found that there is a lot of this contaminant protein in red blood cells, and we also found that it was very abundant in kidney cells. Yet no one studying red blood cells had ever found it, even though it turned out to be astonishingly abundant, there were nearly 200,000 copies per cell. . . . It tends to get your attention."

Agre next asked what red blood cells and renal tubules have in common. Not much, was his first thought. "So I asked a lot of physiologists and cell biologists for suggestions." It was the late John Parker, a membrane physiologist who had been Agre's mentor during his clinical fellowship at UNC, who gave him the clue. "John said to me, 'those are two of the most water permeable tissues in the body. Maybe it's a water channel protein. People have been looking for them for decades.'" Agre tested the hypothesis by microinjecting purified RNA of the purified protein into *Xenopus* eggs. And soon thereafter he was Stockholm bound. Again, two mentors, one a physician-scientist within academe, and one an offsite mentor in industry, prodded Agre to ask the big question, and prepared his mind to follow where the science took him.

Components of a Successful Mentoring Relationship

Much has been written about what constitutes the responsibilities of a mentor. The physician-scientist as mentor has at least six roles to fill: teacher, sponsor, adviser, agent, role model, and confidant. It should also be stressed, however, that the mentor's goal should not be to clone himself or herself. Rather the successful mentor should be an astute enough listener and observer to help the protégé pursue and achieve his or her own dreams. Good mentors need to understand their own limitations and should not be hesitant about encouraging a protégé to seek advice from and follow the examples of others. In fact, one might consider the following roles as the combined responsibilities of a mentoring team of faculty members.

The Mentor as Teacher

As a teacher, the mentor, along with his or her research assistants, trains the protégé in the technical skills unique to their field of research, as well as how to read in an efficient and critical manner and how to reason from first principles. The mentor teaches the fellow how to apply for grants, and reads them critically, several times if necessary.

The Mentor as Sponsor

As sponsor, the mentor introduces the protégé to the critical cast of characters in the trainee's new world. The outstanding mentor is generous with credit when working together, promoting the protégé. When the trainee first presents his or her work, the mentor identifies researchers who have a reputation for helping young people, encouraging the learner to be very open in discussing all aspects of the work, including limitations. The helpful researcher will suggest new experimental approaches. Mentors can help trainees cultivate potential outside support by encouraging "face time" with scholars from other institutions at national meetings and local gatherings. This will prove vital when the time comes to initiate the mentee's academic promotion process.

The successful mentor recommends the protégé for service on grant review study sections of the NIH or other funding agencies. While such an endeavor should warrant hazard pay in the current funding climate, it is vital that young faculty know what actually happens to a grant after it has been submitted. Serving on such review panels will offer the young physician-scientist the opportunity to demonstrate the clarity of his or her scientific reasoning to prominent scholars in the field and learn about general strategies for scientific endeavor; it will help teach the importance of scientific focus and show what constitutes a grant application that receives an outstanding priority score. The generous mentor finds opportunities for the mentee to organize or participate in high-profile conferences and professional societies. I cannot stress enough the intangible but extremely important nature of becoming known to leaders in the field. Once a critical mass of outside experts has become familiar with the protégé's work, that work is more likely to receive a warm reception when such an expert serves as his or her journal or study section reviewer.

The Mentor as Adviser

As adviser, the mentor serves as a sounding board for the trainee to help refine ideas and gain clarity of thought, providing the missing experience. But the seasoned mentor avoids spoon-feeding; there is much to be learned in problem-solving a failed experiment, including a better understanding of the technology, and gaining self-reliance and self-confidence. As adviser, the mentor provides guidance on career choices and the path to promotion, on the need and mechanisms to enhance visibility, and on how to develop leadership skills. The mentor provides feedback on performance or relationships with colleagues and the means of achieving autonomy. One of the key roles of the adviser is to assess how much mentoring and preparatory work the nascent physician-scientist needs. This varies widely with the individual, and is determined by prior training, inherent technical skill, access to appropriate and collegial collaborations, and luck (but with Pasteur's caveat that luck does favor the prepared mind). Among the greatest physician-scientists of our time, Mike Brown and Joe Goldstein argue that the trainee is ready to leave the nest when she or he has acquired technical courage, a sufficient set of skills and the experience and self-confidence to develop new tools when the need arises. As one's science ebbs and flows and turns in all directions, the newly minted physician-scientist embraces the challenge of following the flow of discovery wherever the science leads (Goldstein 1986).

Another mentoring role not yet discussed broadly is that of encouraging the trainee to take risks and set off in new directions. Of course foolhardy risk taking should be avoided, but with a properly honed scientific sense, the benefit is often well worthwhile.

Mike Brown believes it is far too easy to learn one technique and then to repeat essentially the same experiment over and over. "In this fashion one can write many papers, receive large research grants, and remain solidly rooted in the middle of a scientific field. But the true innovator has the confidence to drop one set of experimental crutches and leap to another when he or she must move forward."

The best physician-scientists are agile and recognize when a chance observation, a brainstorm, a concept "borrowed" from another discipline, or new technology offers the possibility of a quantum leap. In my case and that of my colleagues, the successful search for thrombopoietin in our laboratory grew out of an observation borrowed from our colleagues in the oncogene world (Kaushansky 1995). Sequence homology of a novel proto-oncogene, *c-MPL,* and the source of its cDNA cloning, human erythroleukemia cells, suggested to us that it might represent the receptor for the elusive blood platelet growth factor thrombopoietin. This "brainstorm" catalyzed a highly successful collaboration and two years later resulted in the cloning and characterization of thrombopoietin, the primary regulator of platelet production. From this experience we learned that fear of failure could be the death of progress. A research project that appears a totally safe investment has a much smaller chance of making a substantial advance than a project carrying a distinct chance of failure. My fellows are advised to follow the "two-project rule": Choose one project that is of lower risk and very likely to succeed; in baseball parlance, a solid single, or in journal parlance, a first-tier specialty journal article. The second project is chosen so that if successful, the work is attractive to a journal such as *Cell, Science,* or *Nature.* By necessity it is high risk, swinging for a home run, but also running the risk of striking out.

The mentor also serves as the chief academic adviser in all three realms of the physician-scientist domain: research, teaching, and clinical care. Obviously the mentor must be familiar with and be able to explain the departmental, school of medicine, and university criteria, policies, and procedures regarding faculty tracks, reappointment, promotion, and tenure. The mentor advises his or her junior faculty protégé on the criteria for promotion. Specifically he or she will stress the need for a national reputation for outstanding independent scholarship, and how a series of first- or senior-authored peer-reviewed articles in respected journals that tell a coherent story about one's research is the strongest currency in the academic market. Predominant or exclusive participation in scientific groups designed to tackle particularly complex biomedical problems deserves comment here. While biomedical science is increasingly becoming a team sport, at this time not all academic institutions value team contributions to a level sufficient for promotion. At the very minimum, inclusion in such groups as a sole form of academic scholarship should pass the "Would this paper differ significantly if Dr. J. Faculty was not involved in the project?" Given a sufficient number of answers like "There would not have been a paper if Dr. Faculty were not a part of the team" or "The paper would have been published in the *Journal of Obscure Medicine* rather than the *Journal of*

Clinical Investigation if Dr. Faculty had not been part of the group," most (but not all) promotion and tenure committees will be sufficiently convinced to promote Dr. Faculty to associate professor.

A critical ingredient of scientific success is focus. More than anything else, nascent physician-scientists risk losing the kind of focus that requires mental discipline. Without focus, the protégé ends up with numerous unfinished projects. Because time is the most scarce resource in academic life, it is important for mentors to help their mentees master time-management skills. The mentor teaches the fellow to document for himself or herself where the time goes, to spot time-wasting activities and be ruthless in eliminating them.

The scientific mentor is also ideally positioned to advise the protégé on establishing a productive laboratory. For example, during the first year, hiring the best research personnel should take precedence over purchasing the most cutting-edge equipment, and the first order of business should be to get the experimental systems up and running. Knowing how to handle the nitty-gritty, from ordering equipment to hiring postdocs and technicians to recruiting graduate students, can make or break a new faculty member's ability to get up to speed quickly. Competition for graduate students can be intense. Mentors can help mentees make themselves visible to graduate students by encouraging them to do five crucial things.

One is to join at least one affinity group. Crossing departmental and school boundaries, these groups of faculty within biomedical graduate programs focus on common scientific themes, such as vascular biology, inflammation, cancer biology, or stem cells, and can provide the junior faculty member with exposure to a wide range of graduate students in addition to colleagues with whom they may want to collaborate. Another is to give chalk talks at graduate student gatherings. Generally about ten minutes long, these talks provide the young physician-scientist with a forum to "advertise" his or her research to graduate students. Volunteering to teach first-year seminars is also critical. First-year students have not yet committed to an area of research, and the seminar presents an opportune time to reach them. It is also important to cultivate rotation students. When the junior faculty member hosts rotation students, he or she should be encouraged to work with them, to go over papers with them, and talk with them frequently. Finally, it is important for the mentor to help the protégé discover whether there are institutional training (T32) grants he or she can join. Biomedical graduate programs usually maintain a complete list of these training grants, along with their principal investigators.

The mentor should also provide critical advice on growing his or her protégé's science. Once a new faculty member has set his science in motion, he may be tempted to retreat to his office to focus on grant writing. Assuming a positive outcome will be the result, the junior faculty member thus leaves lab projects to graduate students or postdoctoral fellows. Mentors should encourage junior faculty to meet with their own research team members regularly and to monitor the lab's work closely so they can keep pushing it to the next phase. They must help their protégés understand how to troubleshoot as needed, interpret results, and design the next set of experiments. Ultimately, time spent attending to the science will more than pay for itself.

As the young physician-scientist's skills and experience grow, the mentor, in his or her advisory role, must also progressively allow the trainee more and more independence, which is a vital currency in the academic process. Most authors who comment on the topic believe that mentoring is a lifelong process. They argue that input into a trainee's career can extend long after the first NIH R01 grant is secured, as well as after the assistant professorship is attained or even the associate professorship or full professorship. Despite continued input into career decisions, and serving as a scientific sounding board or technical adviser, mentors must avoid hoisting themselves onto the scholarly backs of their protégés. The projects that formed the basis of the mentee's scholarly progress while he or she was in the mentor's laboratory should either be handed over to the trainee or divided into independent units of scientific pursuit for the mentee's and the mentor's laboratories. As the new assistant professor publishes more and more without her mentor as a co-author, her scholarly publications should progressively show less and less of the mentor's fingerprints. To gain academic independence the junior faculty member need not necessarily move away from the mentor's home institution. But generating truly mentor-less publications is essential if the mentor and mentee remain at the same university.

In the realm of teaching, academic progress is highly dependent on outstanding and well-documented educational skills. We have all read faculty manuals commenting that "the candidate should have a record of excellence in teaching students and trainees." The mentor should provide guidance, constructive criticism, and consistent monitoring that targets the protégé's teaching skills, lecture notes, and slide presentations. The mentor should not advise focusing on research to the exclusion of teaching, but should also caution the mentee against taking on major course organization responsibilities.

As faculty manuals often state, "Those who are involved in patient care are expected to be excellent clinicians." If the trainee is going to continue clinical work, which I highly recommend, the mentor should encourage the trainee to become an excellent clinician.

In a survey of over eight thousand clinical and research fellows, instructors, and assistant professors at the Harvard Medical School and its seventeen affiliated hospitals, the mentoring characteristics that were statistically associated with learner satisfaction with a mentor were (1) keeping in touch regarding progress, (2) not abusing power, (3) providing counsel on professional decisions, (4) providing help with building professional networks, (5) providing academic guidance, (6) providing advice relative to career plans and research, and (7) providing opportunities to develop communication skills (Ramanan et al. 2002).

The Mentor as Role Model

As role model, the mentor doesn't just talk the talk but walks the walk. What is on display is the mentor's intellectual and scholarship style. The mentor must unmistakably demonstrate his or her enjoyment of learning and teaching. It does little good for the trainee to be discouraged by continuous complaints about funding, research conditions, or teaching load. "I can't believe I get paid to do this" should replace "I'll never get this grant." The mentor should communicate the thrill of discovery: no drug is more addictive. The best mentors are not always the best teachers, but it certainly helps. Mentoring is the ultimate in teaching because it also involves teaching life lessons. And if the mentor is a clinician, he or she should be an excellent clinician who enjoys the work.

The Mentor as Coach

As coach, the good mentor knows when to offer encouragement, when to push, and when to take a break. The mentor conveys the sense of excitement that is the tool that inspires the trainee to continue along the planned path. When a mentor sets high standards, the fellow is encouraged to achieve full potential: to reach for and achieve more than he or she thought possible. The mentor helps the fellow to take risks, to move outside a zone of comfort. Mentors are invaluable in a search to find the answer to the guiding question about the future: How do you want to be remembered in medicine?

For all nascent physician-scientists a point comes when one asks oneself: "Why pursue the frenetic, intense pace that is academic medicine? Surely a career as a private practice clinician is far less schizophrenic!" Moreover, the literature is replete with articles espousing balance between career and life, arguing that enrichment provided by family, friends, and nonmedical interests or passions deserves equal consideration. Most fellows and junior faculty members in research-intense fields do not see such an idyllic pursuit as compatible with success as a physician-scientist.

And I am forced to agree, even though I recognize that there is disagreement on this point, even among the authors of this book. While having sufficient time for *all* of life's rich experiences is a possible goal for many career paths, except for the most brilliant, it is simply not possible for the physician-scientist. While the quip of a famous former chair of medicine might be a little hyperbolic—"If you can't get it done in twenty-four hours, you will have to work nights"—the truth is that in the world of a physician-scientist, balance between career and other pursuits is often hard to achieve. Nevertheless, my own experience is that a full, rewarding life outside of one's career is possible for a successful physician-scientist. I have been blessed with a rich family life and two intense avocations (one of which is discussed shortly), much enhanced by the work-related travel afforded the physician-scientist.

Each stage of one's career requires a tremendous amount of time and commitment. As a fellow, one has to explore numerous scientific avenues to identify the niche(s) that should be developed into a career. Junior faculty members are writing grants in the time between doing experiments, penning a manuscript, or going to clinic. Middle-level faculty members are working to convince the NIH study section that their research really deserves that all-important second R01 grant, while helping fellows with their K award applications and proofreading their papers and book chapters. Associate professors are taking on an increased teaching load to protect the time their protégés need to develop their own scientific niche, and traveling to study sections and review boards and scientific meetings, where they will attempt to take in both the most exciting scientific findings and the latest clinical advances. Senior faculty members are writing even more grant applications to keep the increased numbers of their group busily occupied with pipette tips and enzymes and mice, drifting over to the "dark side" of administration, serving as an assistant dean, leading an important campus committee, or worst of all chairing a department of medicine.

Part of truthfully coaching the nascent physician-scientist is relaying the immense sense of satisfaction one gains from generating new knowledge. It is helping that young scientist experience the thrill of knowing he or she is the first person on the planet to elucidate a previously confusing element of biology, one that brings important implications to our understanding of human health and disease. It involves helping one's protégé experience the great pleasure that comes with delivering a research talk to colleagues, who thank him for providing the key insight that advances their work. A good coach imparts the sense of amazement that residents express as they finally "get" why you, and now they love to do science in medicine. The inspired mentor counteracts the cynics. The *Journal of the American Medical Association* editorialized that "the highly trained MD-PhD seems out of place in the new primary-care oriented, cost-conscious health care paradigm. If medical schools are to continue to justify dual-degree tracks, they must demonstrate MD-PhDs' contributions to the nation's health care agenda" (Huang 1999). I could not disagree more.

The Mentor as Confidant

As confidant, the mentor is someone the fellow or junior faculty member can talk to, knowing that the discussions are kept in strict confidence. The mentor not only conveys compliments but also points out weaknesses. In writing to his protégé Harvey Cushing, perhaps the most famous physician-scientist of a century ago, Sir William Osler, pointed out the specific aspects of Cushing's behavior that Osler believed would be detrimental to his success. In the letter Osler specifies why this behavior was a problem, and ends by relating his certainty that Cushing would not mind the criticism but would understand that Osler had his protégé's interests at heart. Painting a truthful picture of a career as a physician-scientist is one of the most important roles for a mentor. For the physician-scientist with a basic science orientation, this includes a candid assessment of the protégé's laboratory skills.

Institutional Mentoring: Level-Specific Enhancements to Nurture the (Nascent) Physician-Scientist

In addition to supporting the responsibilities of individual mentors, there is much that an institution can and should provide to aid in the development of physician-scientists, both to kindle the flame that leads the bright and energetic learner toward this career pathway and to encourage those who have already seen the light. Because of the competing demands of scientific rigor and clinical excellence, of becoming bilingual (my term for speaking the languages of science and of clinical medicine), the pathway toward success as a physician-scientist is already strewn with numerous hurdles. We must collectively find a way to lessen the size of the boulders in our young people's path.

Mentoring Internal Medicine Residents

Residency is an ideal time to inculcate trainees in clinical investigation. This was well illustrated in a survey of the 138 internal medicine residents at Johns Hopkins School of Medicine, which described the value of such a program (Rivera, Levine, and Wright 2005). About half of the respondents to the survey presented a clinical vignette and half a research abstract. Residents participated in research for a variety of reasons, including intellectual curiosity (73 percent), career development (60 percent), and as a way to fulfill a mandatory scholarly activity requirement of their residency program (32 percent). The most common barriers to complete satisfaction were insufficient time (79 percent), inadequate research skills (45 percent), and lack of a research curriculum (44 percent). Residents who had presented research abstracts devoted more time to their projects than those who exhibited clinical vignettes. Sixty-nine percent of residents thought research should be a residency requirement.

With a goal of exciting the nascent "late bloomer" physician-scientist, and mindful of Dan Foster's admonition that "the physician/scientist must become more visible to our learners to convey the excitement of the discovery of new knowledge," the Department of Medicine at the University of California, San Diego, has instituted an "inculcation in the science of medicine" program. The chair and physician-scientist "teaching attendings" present illustrative patients and lead a Socratically based science in medicine discussion with the medical students, interns, and residents at each morning report. Also included in the program is a curriculum that teaches the skills of patient-oriented research in which all residents deliver monthly evidence-based reviews on topics of clinical relevance. The highlight of the program occurs in the second or third year of residency, when approximately two-thirds of our class spends two to three months of protected time conducting biomedical research of broad scope. The titles of the projects presented in our inaugural year included "N-Glycolylneuarminic Acid, a Common Mammalian Sialic Acid No Longer Endogenously Produced by Man," "Assessment of Coronary Flow Reserve Using Myocardial Contrast Echocardiography," "The Purification of Surfactant Protein D and Development of an ELISA for Measuring Levels in Bronchoalveolar Lavage Fluid," and "p38 MAPK Expression and Phosphorylation in Human Tissues: Modulation by Insulin, Obesity, and Type 2 Diabetes Mellitus." Of the nine participating residents, at this writing six are assistant professors in academic departments. Over the first five years, seventy-seven residents participated in research blocks with topics of study very similar to those in our initial year. As physician-scientists concerned with human health and disease, the leaders of our department believe we are in a particularly favorable position to foster the first step in expanding the pipeline of physicians into the scholarly realm, the scientific seduction.

Mentoring during Fellowship and Postdoctoral Training

For most physician-scientists, especially "late bloomers," fellowship, and extension of this training into a postdoctoral fellowship, a period I commonly refer to as "academic purgatory," is the critical period that will often not only launch a career but also define its scientific landscape for the following twenty to thirty years. With the difficulty in financially supporting this group of individuals, as evidenced by the decline in NIH-sponsored T32 training grants, this critical period in the spawning of the physician-scientist is particularly vulnerable. Providing a rich academic environment in which our fellows can flourish is becoming increasingly essential to expanding the physician-scientist pipeline and repairing its leaks. The common denominator of postdoctoral training is the laboratory clinical research group meeting, the rigor of which is dependent on the primary mentor. But there are enhancements to the scientific environment that institutions can and should supplement. Medical specialty–based clinical case conferences should be offered. In addition, there should be a rich selection of scientifically based weekly seminars. In these, faculty and senior fellows from the subspecialty division and related disciplines would present ongoing laboratory work, highlight the science of medicine, and illustrate how different physician-scientists approach the myriad of scientific challenges identified by their clinical colleagues. Such seminars provide an outstanding communications opportunity to give incoming fellows a look at available mentors and their teaching skills.

Although the diversity of career interests of physician-scientists is among the richest in all of biomedicine, there are several common elements to the training of those who seek a career as a physician-scientist. Fellowship is an ideal time to provide rigorous training in these common elements.

Ethics Mentoring

An analysis of a national survey of over 7,700 early and mid-level biomedical and social science researchers who received research support from the NIH found that there was a strong inverse relationship between receipt of separate or integrated training in research ethics or mentoring related to ethics, and ethically problematic behavior (Anderson, Horn, and Risbey 2007). Based on this and several other similar studies, the NIH now mandates ethics training as part of sponsored fellowship programs.

Academic Skills Mentoring

The lifeblood of our profession is communication. Public speaking comes easily to some and less easily to others. But the successful physician-scientist must be able to communicate effectively in order to flourish. If the fruits of their labor are to be appropriately translated into clinical progress, physician-scientists must be able to communicate their innovative translational ideas to grant review study sections and the results of their findings to scientific and clinical colleagues. Rather than leaving the development of such proficiencies to the "see one–do one–teach one" model, or to chance, research-intense institutions should strongly consider providing seminars on academic skills. The "How to Give a Talk" talk, the "How to Write a Grant" seminar, and the "How to Negotiate a Job" discussion are examples of such institutional mentoring.

Mentoring Junior Faculty

While officially academically independent, the newly minted, recently appointed physician-scientist faculty member deserves much attention. Increasingly, such individuals have not yet received their first NIH R01 or equivalent award (the average age of a first R01 being forty-two years) or developed the collaborations that will further enhance their productivity and impact. Nor have they been mentored on how to mentor, which is a skill that junior faculty eager to build their laboratories with graduate students and postdoctoral fellows will need to master. There are many opportunities for the institution to step in and enhance the new assistant professor's prospects for promotion on time or sooner.

Organized Mentoring Programs

Several universities now offer organized mentoring programs to improve the tools of junior faculty members and provide them with academic survival skills. One nationwide program is the National Center for Leadership in Academic Medicine (NCLAM). A report from the NCLAM program at the University of California, San Diego (UCSD), School of Medicine illustrates the advantages of providing a combination of didactic information and mentored guidance in developing a research plan (Wingard, Garman, and Reznik 2004). Among sixty-seven participants in the program, 85 percent remained at UCSD one to five years later, 93 percent of whom remained in academic medicine. Their confidence in skills needed for academic success improved. In comparison to the results of the same survey instrument administered prior to the nine-month course, 53 percent noted improved personal leadership skills, 19 percent improved in research, 33 percent improved in teaching, and 76 percent improved in administration skills. Given the financial information provided and the improved retention rates compared to historical controls, the savings in recruitment were greater than the costs of the program. Additional coursework opportunities are also available at many research-intense medical schools. For example, at UCSD we have created the Clinical Research Education through Supplemental Training (CREST) program, funded through an NIH K12 grant. Through this program junior faculty members can obtain training in biostatistics, governmental regulatory bodies, clinical trial design, and several other courses individually; when the training is taken to completion, they can obtain a master's in advanced study degree.

In addition to local programs to help mentor junior faculty members, professional societies are increasingly providing training programs in clinical and translational research approaches and methods, using intensive mentoring strategies. For example, the American Society of Hematology (ASH) offers the Clinical Research Training Institute (CRTI), a year-long program kicked off with a week of concentrated didactic sessions and mentoring, using the learners' own research proposals, with a faculty-to-learner ratio of 1:1 or greater. Over the ensuing year the mentors periodically discuss progress, hurdles, and their solutions with their trainees. Five years of CRTI graduates are being evaluated to assess the impact of the ASH program. The American Society of Clinical Oncology and American Association for Cancer Research jointly, and the American Society for Blood and Marrow Transplantation, have also created similar programs.

Creating Rich Research Neighborhoods

Another vital role for the institution is to facilitate the formation of productive scientific groups. While academic fanfare is often reserved for individual accomplishments, mobilizing teams of talented physician-scientists as well as others with complementary skill sets is the most effective way to solve the complex biomedical problems that face our world. Sir James Black, the Scottish physician who left academics and joined the pharmaceutical industry to create β-blockers (e.g., propranolol) and the histamine-2 antagonists (e.g., cimetidine), has stated that the majority of significant research discoveries result from "the concentrated efforts of small teams of talented and highly focused scientists."

Young physician-scientists are well advised to join a thematic research group, which will become their scientific support network. The group may be large or small, but should be "real"—not assembled merely to acquire funding. And the groups ought to be in close geographical proximity. Despite the marvels of electronic communication, there is no substitute for running into a colleague in the hallway and discussing a scientific problem. For example, if a hematology laboratory studies hematopoietic growth factor signaling, it makes far more sense for it to be adjacent to rheumatologists studying tumor necrosis factor signaling, or endocrinologists studying insulin signaling, than to another hematology group studying hemoglobin.

Mentoring "Offsite"

Under certain circumstances it is wiser for the trainee to obtain specialized scientific training from individuals or groups outside his or her usual divisional or departmental setting. This road less traveled can lead to numerous dividends. For example, I learned how to build cDNA libraries and clone genes at a (then) small biotechnology company. In addition to providing an excellent learning environment, it allowed me to establish several valuable scientific relationships, which a few years later led to an important collaboration in the cloning of thrombopoietin. One study found that placing pediatric fellows and junior faculty members in non-pediatric departments during periods of training enhances much-needed multidisciplinary ties among several medical school departments (Rivkees and Genel 2007). While this offsite mentoring model can be extremely rewarding, under certain circumstances it can lead to a sense of isolation for the junior faculty member, or drift in purpose. Although the offsite mentor can be outstanding at providing scientific guidance, it is usually the home division or department mentor who best understands the career perspective needed to remain on a successful physician-scientist pathway.

Financial Support for the Nascent Physician-Scientist

It is imperative that our junior faculty believe there is institutional support for their work. In the current NIH funding climate, this translates into the kind of fiscal security that will allow an assistant professor to establish his or her scientific program without the need to perform an inappropriate amount of clinical work to generate salary. Street wisdom suggests that the "start-up" package for a newly minted assistant professor involved in laboratory research is from $500,000 to $1 million (to cover salary, equipment, personnel, and other research expenses for the first three years). While serving as chair of a research-intensive department of medicine, I have found that such guidelines are of little importance. What is critical is giving the new assistant professor the personalized resources that will maximize the likelihood of his or her success. For a new faculty member who wants to establish a proteomics program using mass spectroscopy, for example, the start-up costs for equipment alone will clearly exceed those required by a colleague who needs only a tissue culture hood, immunofluorescence antibodies, and access to an already available confocal microscopy facility.

In addition to university funds, most professional societies, such as the American Society of Hematology, the American Heart Association, and the American Society for Clinical Oncology, offer moderate levels of support for promising postdoctoral fellows and junior faculty members. Institutions, including their clinical departments, should also contribute to the development of junior faculty members, particularly during times of transition. For example, the University of Kentucky offers a three-year, $75,000 per year grant to support assistant professors who are working toward obtaining a K08 award (University of Kentucky 2008). To help them attain a first R01 (or equivalent) grant, the UCSD Department of Medicine offers four $50,000 per year grants to junior faculty members who are completing a K08 (or equivalent) award. A study of the likelihood of remaining in academics (Weinert et al. 2006) found that the perceived likelihood of pulmonary and critical care fellows and junior faculty entering or remaining in an academic career was greatest for individuals with institutional research support.

Academic Oversight

In order to help plug the leaky physician-scientist career pipeline, no junior faculty member should be left behind. The department chair or institute director should interview new faculty members annually for at least five years to address their concerns and ensure that proper mentorship is in place. While several academic institutions advocate the formal assignment of mentors to new faculty members, most research-intense programs forgo the "arranged marriage" model for a number of reasons. One significant problem is that senior faculty who are pressured into becoming mentors may be uninterested in and unhelpful to the protégés assigned to them. The institution should therefore provide help to junior faculty members so they can identify appropriate mentors. This will be especially important for individuals who are new to their university. The department chair or center director can screen faculty as mentors, verifying that the potential mentor is willing to spend the necessary time and accept the responsibility of mentoring. He or she can remind the potential mentor that having a trainee is a responsibility and a privilege, not a right. The department should also help determine if a potential mentor has adequate research expertise, resources, and experience for a particular learner.

Once the mentors for new fellows and faculty are identified, the institution has additional responsibilities. This includes careful monitoring of the mentoring process. The problematic mentor-mentee partnership must be avoided, or at least detected early and remedied. Many of these conflicts are due to possessive mentors who do not encourage or permit rapid enough independence. It has been my experience that the overly possessive mentor needs a visit to the department chair's office to help clarify his or her goals.

Monitoring Physician-Scientist Mentoring

If the institution seeks to enhance the training and development of physician-scientists, like all interventions in biomedicine, the mentoring experience should be measured. First, the program should state the goals of the mentoring program. Most programs would consider the following the sine qua non of a successful program:

1. New faculty will gain a clearer sense of the rigors and rewards of a career as a physician-scientist.
2. New faculty will acquire a better awareness of expectations for academic advancement.
3. New faculty will develop rapport with one or preferably many additional colleagues.
4. The duration of the transition period from new investigator to established researcher will decrease.
5. Career satisfaction of new physician-scientists should improve.

Therefore some suggested metrics include:

1. Reduced numbers of individuals transferring from tenure track to clinical track at the mid-career review.
2. Increased numbers of successful assistant to associate professor promotions.
3. Reduced mean duration of time spent as an assistant professor.
4. Increased numbers of NIH K (or equivalent) and R (or equivalent) awards to faculty members.
5. Increased medical student, resident, and fellow interest in biomedical research on *anonymous* exit surveys of career goals.

Alternate Mentoring Models

The notion of a senior professional promoting the career of a junior protégé has shaped the development of mentoring programs in academic medicine and other fields for over a century, with senior physicians modeling desired behaviors and attitudes for their juniors (Pololi and Knight 2005). Proponents of alternate mentoring systems suggest that rather than relying on a dyadic relationship, a group process characterized by non-hierarchical peer relationships, protégé empowerment, and self-direction has a number of advantages. These authors argue that a reflective process that involves the self-identification of personal and professional goals that are consistent with an individual's personal values is far more likely to result in career satisfaction than the classic model of one-on-one, senior-to-junior mentoring.

Responsibilities of the Trainee

Mentoring is a two-way street, with mentors needing trainees as much as trainees need a mentor (Baughman et al. 2008). As with all teaching, mentors often learn as much or more from pupils than they teach them. A researcher gets more done by involving bright young people on projects than working as a lone wolf. The mentor benefits from the reflected glory of the trainee who does well. But the major benefit is the fun of interacting with young people—what Osler termed "the greatest zest in life"—and the satisfaction of perpetuating the species. Nevertheless, mentoring relationships take work, on the part of both mentor and mentee. Without that effort, the experience can have a negative impact on one or both individuals. The previous discussion focused on the responsibilities of the mentor, both individual and institutional; but the trainee also has responsibilities. In order to optimize the training relationship, trainees should commit to (1) assuming responsibility for their career; (2) asking for and accepting advice and constructive criticism; (3) becoming familiar with their departmental, school, and university criteria, policies, and procedures regarding faculty tracks, reappointment, promotion, and tenure; (4) continuing to add to the knowledge base in their areas of expertise; (5) developing a professional network which includes both those recommended by the mentor and those personally identified; (6) maintaining the confidentiality of the relationship; (7) striving for academic excellence in all fields of expertise; and (8) providing ongoing evidence of productivity, particularly in the area of publications and teaching.

Nascent physician-scientists should also take care in choosing a mentor. Besides expertise in the scientific field and teaching skills, other, less obvious traits that augur well for a productive relationship are the capacity of the mentor (1) to manage and organize his or her research group; (2) to display a reputation for setting high standards in a congenial atmosphere; and (3) to be fiscally secure, at least for three to four years, an average amount of time for the mentee to begin to gain independence. Mentees should do their due diligence in selecting a mentor by speaking with present and former advisees and gaining personal impressions through face-to-face interviews.

A key question for such discussions is whether a particular mentor's style is compatible with the trainee's personality. At the risk of great oversimplification, there are two types of mentors: "short-leash" and "long-leash."

The short-leash mentor will help plan each day's experiments, frequently discuss the results with the learner, and, by having a vision of how the work should proceed, prevent the mentee from going astray. The advantage to this approach is that there is less chance that the mentee will fall into the cracks, lose direction, or make many errors. The long-leash mentor, by contrast, will always be available for discussion, advice, technical consultation, or demonstration, but will allow the trainee to design, execute, and interpret his or her own experiments. The advantage to this approach is that the mentee can be very productive and gain a great deal of self-confidence—that is, run with the leash. The risk is that the mentee will go astray, thus potentially strangling on it. Given these divergent approaches, it behooves trainees to consider which style of learning they are most comfortable with, and choose the mentor accordingly.

The advisee should also have realistic expectations of his or her mentor. Advisers are only human, and one's mentor also has his or her own career to advance. The mentee should optimize communication. For example, if the mentor travels a great deal, make appointments. Trainees should be efficient and organized in their interactions with their mentor. It is often helpful to have an agenda or list of topics and questions for discussion. After the meeting, agreements should be summarized. When requesting review of creative work, the advisee should not submit a rough draft to the mentor for input. The work should be well organized and free of typographical errors. After reworking a manuscript or proposal, the trainee should highlight the changed sections so that the mentor does not have to reread the entire paper. Criticism should be accepted graciously. It is the mentor's job to evaluate objectively the trainee's work and progress. While there may be disagreements, the trainee should at least consider the adviser's opinions. If, after further reflection, disagreements persist, it is crucial for the trainee again to discuss and rationally defend his or her position.

In this chapter I have illustrated the approaches that one physician-scientist has found to be successful in mentoring, and how a department of medicine at one medical school approaches fixing the leaky career pipeline of physician-scientists. There are currently more than 120 medical schools in the United States. The old adage "If you have seen one medical school, you have seen one medical school" is particularly appropriate for the subject of mentoring physician-scientists. While I have formulated the collective ideas expressed in this chapter over nearly a quarter-century as a faculty member at two research-intense schools of medicine, the University of Washington and University of California, San Diego, they have also been informed by a widespread network of outstanding mentors and colleagues. No discussion of mentoring of physician-scientists would be complete without mention of one's own mentors: Clem Finch, who convinced me that there was more science in hematology than in any other discipline; John Adamson and Earl Davie, my dual fellowship mentors, who taught me scientific, clinical, and academic rigor; my many graduate students, postdoctoral fellows, and close collaborators, without whom my science would never have gone so far; and my family, Lauren, Alexis, and Joshua, who have witnessed firsthand the energy, effort, and zeal necessary to develop a career as a late bloomer physician-scientist, espouse its virtues, and walk the walk of this unique lifestyle.

11

Mentoring the Physician-Scientist

A DEVELOPMENTAL APPROACH

Alan L. Schwartz, MD, PhD,
and Margaret K. Hostetter, MD

Mentoring future physician-scientists involves the identification, recruitment, and retention of those who have the potential to become the successful investigators of the next generation. Therefore it is essential to encourage the participation of junior and senior physician-scientist faculty members—potential future mentors—in such medical student activities as combined MD-PhD degree Medical Scientist Training Programs (MSTPs), first- and second-year student teaching activities, and special programs for students considering research careers.

These "cultivation" activities should complement time spent in specialty education. Wright and colleagues (1998) found that role models identified by internal medicine residents at four institutions consistently spent more than 25 percent of their time teaching and devoted more than twenty-five hours per week to teaching and conducting rounds while serving as attending physicians.

The recruitment of potential physician-scientists should emphasize those aspects of a research career that are attractive to today's generation of students, as discussed in chapter 6 by Ann Brown. Because today's medical school classes are equally divided between male and female students, medical school leaders should recognize that the flexibility of an academic research career, particularly as it relates to its potential to accommodate work-family balance, is a "marketable" aspect. Students and residents often fail to understand that the apparent eight-to-nine-hour day of an office-based clinical practice is extended by unpredictably busy night and

weekend on-call responsibilities that are typically divided equally among
the practitioners. For physician-scientists in most academic subspecialties,
however, night and weekend clinical requirements constitute no more than
a one- or two-month commitment per year. In addition, academic maternity and paternity leaves are typically paid and frequently more generous
in length than in clinical practice. At many institutions the tenure clock
can be stopped for up to one year after the birth of a child. Establishment
of child care centers on campus and sliding scales for fees are attractive
potential benefits for young investigators, whose salaries may initially
fall below those of peers who have entered private practice or who focus
purely on clinical work.

Retention of physician-scientists must emphasize clarity of expectations for promotion, continued monitoring of progress, and the provision
of successful role models. Given the scarcity of women in top academic
positions (fewer than 10 percent of department chairs and 15 percent of
professors across all medical disciplines), the need for female role models
outstrips the supply (Ley and Hamilton 2008). Nevertheless, the mentor
should make every effort to point out examples of gender-based success
and to encourage the trainee to observe how these faculty members balance work and family responsibilities.

Mentoring the future physician-scientist therefore requires a flexible
approach that we believe should be keyed to the developmental stage of the
trainee, from medical student through appointment to the junior faculty and
beyond. In this chapter we focus on each stage of the physician-scientist's
career trajectory, identify the professional and personal issues which affect
that progression, and provide examples of mentoring programs that have
proved successful at each stage of development (see table 11.1).

For illustrative purposes we have selected several pediatric mentoring
programs because each emphasizes one key aspect of this process and because each of these models has been successful to date. We believe that
these examples are applicable to mentoring not only academic pediatricians but also physician-scientists in general. Finally, we conclude with
several points of self-reflection for the future, including our view of significant challenges.

History of the Physician-Scientist: Early Beginnings

The history of the physician-scientist is long and broad and spiced with
colorful characters and illustrative developments. It is addressed in depth
in chapter 1 by Andrew Schafer. In pediatrics, the history of formal mentoring of the physician-scientist is over a century old. One might define the

Table 11.1. Developmental mentoring strategies

Rank	Approach	Components
Medical student	Informal	Summer research experience; observation
MSTP student	Formal	Thesis committee; defined curriculum
	Informal	Research mentorship; scientific networks
Resident	Formal	Research paths in residency
	Informal	Exposure to investigators as physicians on the wards
Fellow	Formal	Appointed research mentor; scholarly oversight committee; defined curriculum; published scholarship
	Informal	Scientific networks
Junior faculty	Formal	Annual goal setting with section chief or chair; annual/biannual faculty development reviews
	Informal	Faculty mentors; departmental or sectional retreats

founding of the American Pediatric Society in 1887 as a landmark event for pediatrics to emerge as a field separate from medicine and obstetrics. There were few "academic" pediatricians at that time, among them Abraham Jacobi and L. Emmett Holt in New York. Job Lewis Smith led a small group of colleagues to establish the American Pediatric Society in order to focus on the study of diseases of children and for the promotion of pediatric education and research. Jacobi was selected as the first president of the organization.

Arguably the first pediatric physician-scientist was John Howland (1873–1926). First as chair of pediatrics at Washington University in St. Louis and thereafter at Johns Hopkins Medical School, Howland organized, built, and directed the first modern, scientifically based department of pediatrics in the United States. This included a fully equipped biochemistry laboratory within the children's hospital. His trainees—Park, Powers, Marriott, Gamble, and Davidson—became pediatric physician-scientist luminaries in their own right and carried the mentor-mentee role into the next generation. Today's pediatric physician-scientists can trace their professional lineage in large part to Howland and his trainees.

Medical Students

In order to address the clinical focus of most medical students who are not enrolled in combined MD-PhD MSTP programs, mentoring at this stage often derives from contact with faculty role models in a clinical setting.

Short-term research experiences that evolve from a clinical question can be a powerful influence in recruiting medical students to careers as physician-scientists. The opportunity to participate in a relevant, often patient-related research project for a short period of time (e.g., summer break) often leads to longer and more intense research experiences. In addition, the opportunity to observe physician-scientists as they move between laboratory, clinical activities, and family roles seems to provide an intensely personal and meaningful experience that amplifies the more traditional role of the physician as clinician.

One example of medical student involvement in research is the thesis requirement at some medical schools. A drawback is that this often requires as much as an additional year added to the traditional four-year curriculum.

National Summer Research Program

The National Summer Research Program for Medical Students begun by the American Pediatric Society and the Society for Pediatric Research in 1991 represents another approach. This program was designed specifically to enable students to participate in a research opportunity in an institution other than the medical school they attend. Students in this program, who are paid a stipend, spend approximately three months working under the supervision of an experienced scientist (generally a pediatric physician-scientist) in one of the over three hundred participating laboratories conducting pediatric research. Applications are solicited from students at all medical schools in the United States, and evaluated by a steering committee, which selects the top students and matches them by location and mentor. The program, which has funding that is sufficient to support approximately fifty students each year, has received over two thousand applications, and at this writing almost seven hundred students have participated in it. The program has successfully attracted highly qualified, ethnically and racially diverse medical students. It has also engaged the contributions of world-class pediatric physician-scientists as mentors for these students. It thus represents a highly productive and cost-effective mechanism to expose future physicians to the opportunities and challenges of careers as pediatric scientists. Past trainees have entered pediatric residencies at three times the national average.

MSTP Trainees

The Medical Scientist Training Program (MSTP), established by the National Institutes of Health in 1964, offers students an integrated program of graduate training in the biomedical sciences and clinical training offered through medical schools, fulfilling the requirements for combined MD-PhD degrees. The PhD mentoring experience is central to the MSTP philosophy. Its goals are the development of critical thinking and technical competence, the completion of a meaningful body of research, and the establishment of a foundation for a continued career in science. Other benefits include the day-to-day contact with a well-funded scientist, physician or not, and the opportunity for networking that is a critical underpinning of collaborative research.

Since the first combined MD-PhD programs began, they have provided training to thousands of students. Through the decades the program has continued to grow in distinction, quality, and quantity. The MSTP supports the training of students with outstanding credentials and the potential to undertake careers in biomedical research and academic medicine. By 2009 there were forty NIH-funded MSTP programs with over nine hundred trainees, with approximately 170 positions available each year. In addition, about seventy-five medical schools that do not have NIH-funded MSTP programs also offer combined MD-PhD degree training. In 1998 the NIH surveyed MD-PhD graduates since 1975 and found that 84 percent of those from NIH-funded MSTP programs and 68 percent of graduates of non-NIH-funded combined MD-PhD degree programs were currently in academia. Roy Silverstein and Paul DiCorleto further explore the combined degree programs in chapter 9, which addresses the relationship between MD and PhD scientists in medical research.

In terms of attracting students specifically to pediatric careers, the national MSTP data (1976–2002) reveal that approximately 15 percent of 1976–1995 graduates and 13 percent of 1996–2002 graduates entered careers in pediatrics. In an independent survey Brian Sullivan at Washington University School of Medicine in 2002 compared graduates (1976–2002) from twenty NIH-funded MSTP programs with those from nineteen non-NIH-funded MD-PhD programs. He found that 14 percent of the MSTP graduates and 18 percent of the non-NIH-funded MD-PhD graduates entered pediatrics. Unfortunately there are no national data as to the career outcomes of these trainees, particularly relating to long-term career successes in research.

Residency and Fellowship

Because MSTP initiatives have been considered largely successful, other programs to recruit and train physician-scientists either immediately before or just after residency have adopted similar mentoring approaches.

Pediatric Scientist Development Program

The Pediatric Scientist Development Program (PSDP), funded for over twenty years by the National Institute of Child Health and Human Development (NICHD) of the NIH and a consortium of private foundations, uses the inspiration of disease encountered during the residency years to recruit MDs in their third year of residency. The program supports an intensive two- to three-year basic, translational or clinical research experience under the mentorship of outstanding scientists in the United States or Canada after completion of the clinical fellowship years.
The hallmarks of the PSDP are:

1. The focus is multi-institutional, in contrast to the local focus of NIH institutional (T32) training grants. A candidate may be nominated from one institution as a resident and elect to do his or her research at another as a fellow.
2. For those candidates proposing basic research projects, two years of research experience are not interrupted by clinical responsibilities.
3. Candidates are encouraged to seek a research experience beyond the walls of the department of pediatrics. Most PSDP trainees perform research outside the pediatric department in the laboratories of basic science or other clinical departments. This has two advantages: the fellow is not confined to the more limited scope of research available in pediatric sections, and the basic science laboratory benefits from the clinical insight of the fellow (Hostetter 2002).

The program emphasizes both formal and informal mentoring:

Formal

- Supervision of the overall research and career development of the individual trainee by the laboratory chief, most often outside the department of pediatrics.
- Annual meetings with the PSDP steering committee for career development seminars and programmatic evaluation.

Informal

- Day-to-day mentoring in the laboratory by identified laboratory personnel.
- Collegial mentoring by members of the PSDP steering committee, who serve as sounding boards for career decisions during fellowship and transition to faculty status. Oftentimes these relationships continue well into the faculty years.

Career development is emphasized at annual meetings, with focused workgroups dedicated to common training issues. For example, incoming fellows and those in their first year of the PSDP discuss such topics as how to work with a mentor. Trainees in years two and three may engage with faculty in panel discussions on negotiating the first faculty position. The program actively encourages networking among fellows and laboratories. Of eighty-nine trainees who entered the program between 1987 and 2000, at this writing thirty-four are principal investigators (PI) on more than sixty R-, P-, or U-level awards from the NIH, and two have PI status in Canada. Thus 40 percent of the trainees have attained funding from the NIH or Canadian Institutes of Health Research (CIHR) at the level of independent investigator. Interestingly, MD trainees with three years of training in the PSDP compete just as successfully for independent investigator status on NIH awards as do their MD-PhD counterparts.

Just as with graduate students concluding their PhD work, the medical fellow faces the need to negotiate for the first faculty position at the end of the fellowship. Mentoring efforts directed toward these decisions are especially well received. The ability of PSDP trainees to take advantage of physician-scientists who are outside the departments of pediatrics does not hinder their return to the department; indeed, of 120 trainees, only eight are no longer in academic pediatrics. Assignment of a member of the PSDP steering committee as an informal mentor ensures that the trainee has an extrainstitutional perspective to inform his or her decisions and provides a reservoir of experience that can be extremely useful to the young faculty recruit.

Scholarship Oversight Committees

In recent years the American Board of Pediatrics in concert with a variety of interested organizations, including those representing the subspecialties and under the auspices of the Federation of Pediatric Organizations, brought forward new guidelines for scholarly training activities during subspecialty education (see, e.g., Balistreri et al. 2006). Among the newer paradigms are the expanded pathways for combining general and subspecialty pediatric training (described earlier in this chapter), the requirement of written scholarly work during subspecialty training, and the American Board of Pediatrics–mandated establishment of a three-member scholarship oversight committee for assistance, supervision, and verification of the scholarly activity of the trainee. The scholarship oversight committee serves to evaluate the suitability of the scholarly pursuit, determine the course of action, and ensure successful completion of the project. It also functions much like a thesis committee for a predoctoral candidate.

The required diversity of the scholarship oversight committee broadens the fellow's network and also serves to provide advocacy, informal advising, and accessible role models. Furthermore, in order to minimize real or apparent conflicts of interest, the subspecialty fellowship program director is not expected to serve as a standing member of the scholarship oversight committee.

Junior Faculty

At the time of appointment to the junior faculty position, mentoring goals are typically directed toward faculty development and retention. The young faculty member must understand the promotional tracks at his or her institution, the track for which he or she is being groomed, as well as the criteria and timeline for promotion. The junior faculty member should also understand the organization and governance of the academic institution and the various routes to obtain intrainstitutional resources. Access to graduate students is crucial for young physician-scientists who are trying to establish their own independent research programs. Clarity regarding the need for secondary appointments in a graduate department, as well as departmental service requirements (teaching, interviewing, serving on thesis committees of trainees and other laboratories), must be provided. Access to core facilities is often another important component of success. Mentoring physician-scientists as they make the transition to junior faculty status should clearly address not only these needs but also the composition and structure of the total institutional package that will support the research program of the novice physician-scientist.

Non-academic goals most often center on balancing personal and professional activities. Junior faculty are typically appointed just as they are starting families and their children are old enough to leave the home for a preschool setting. Access to top-tier day care facilities that accommodate the often demanding schedules of physician-scientists is a powerful recruiting tool for candidates of both genders. Flexibility in timing of the tenure decision for women in their childbearing years is equally important for both PhD and MD scientists.

NIH-Funded Child Health Research Centers

A critical stage in one's development as a physician-scientist is the transition from subspecialty fellow to emerging junior faculty member. The former's time is largely protected, while the latter often lacks adequate resources, time, direction, and mentorship. The Child Health Research Centers were established to address these issues. The Child Health Research

Center (CHRC) program emerged through congressional action taken in response to efforts by the Pediatric Research Societies (Society for Pediatric Research and American Pediatric Society) and the National Association of Children's Hospitals. The goal of the program, which relies on the Child Health Research Career Development Award, is to establish "Centers of Excellence" in pediatric research that provide basic science training for pediatricians who have completed their subspecialty training.

Funding began in 1990 with the support of six centers and increased to nineteen centers by 1992 through an NIH K12 award mechanism. This program provides the background, techniques, and tools that junior investigator-scholars need to perform translational research and to secure independent research funding. In each center, established investigator-mentors provide expertise and make their laboratory facilities available to junior investigator-scholars for research projects that will enhance the scholars' basic science research skills. This experience also enables the scholars to generate preliminary data that can be included in grant applications for independent funding.

During the first seventeen years of the program, the NICHD funded over six hundred junior pediatric physician-scientists scholars, working in fourteen different subspecialty areas of pediatrics, in thirty pediatric departments throughout the United States. Within this group there were by 2007 eighteen tenured professors and eighty tenure-track associate professors. Overall, one-fourth of the scholars had been successful in obtaining NIH R-level (independent) funding (see table 11.2). In the most successful centers, 80 percent of the scholars had obtained NIH funding (R, U, and K awards).

While successful in several areas, these centers as a whole have fallen short of their overall goals in some specific important ones. Why had only 67 percent of trainees applied for independent NIH awards? Is a 26 percent

Table 11.2. CHRC Scholars' (1990–2007) NIH Grant Application and Success Rates

Total CHRC scholars tracked	617
Person NIH applications* submitted	415
Person NIH applications rate	67%
Person NIH funding success	308
Person NIH funding rate	74%
Overall person NIH funding rate	50%
Overall person R01 funding rate	26%

Source: Courtesy K. Winer, NICHD.
*Total NIH applications = 2478

overall person R01 funding rate a success story? The 67 percent independent NIH award application rate represents that of the entire 617 trainees
over the first seventeen years of the program. Institution-to-institution
variation is high, with some individual centers having application rates exceeding 90 percent. The 26 percent overall person R01 funding rate, while
better than the rate for all new investigators during these years (1990–
2007), is less than that of the Pediatric Scientist Development Program.
Again, there is marked center-to-center variation, with several centers
having rates exceeding 50 percent. This raises several questions. Should
there be fewer centers? Should a higher bar be set for funding competing
renewals? Should new centers demonstrate a track record of success prior
to selection? What is the role of the mentors for these trainees? These issues
might form the basis for programmatic redefinition.

Organizational Structure, Governance, and Cultural Awareness

Each academic medical center has evolved over time with its own culture, organizational structure, governance, and a multitude of idiosyncrasies. The organizational structure and governance are essential for all
faculty, especially junior faculty, to understand. This structure will define
the responsibilities and authorities of the building blocks of the academic
center (departments, divisions, institutes, centers) and the interrelation-
ships among them. Organizational structure and governance also define
who has which resources and how they can be accessed. Mentors experienced in understanding the organizational structure and governance
can help their mentees by knowing where the resources are and how to
engage them.

One case in point is access to graduate students. In many academic medical centers, graduate students are restricted to training for their PhD only
in the laboratories of faculty within the department that grants the PhD
degree. A mentor who understands this requirement and creates opportunities for his or her mentee to be introduced to that department paves
the way for the young physician-scientist to have graduate students train
in his or her laboratory. A "secondary" appointment in a basic science department, as described earlier, often comes with additional responsibilities
including teaching graduate or medical school courses, serving on thesis
committees of trainees in other laboratories, service on other committees,
engagement in support of training grants, and interviewing prospective
graduate students and faculty candidates. By and large these issues of department "citizenship," while potentially time-consuming for the junior
faculty member, can be richly rewarding. They provide an opportunity to

meet a broad array of creative minds, explore new avenues of thought, develop new collegial relations, nucleate new ideas, and potentially attract new graduate students to one's laboratory.

In addition, the physician-scientist based in a clinical department (e.g., pediatrics) brings a wealth of resources to the basic science department (e.g., developmental biology): access to colleagues across the disciplines of pediatric medicine, access to patients and patient-derived materials for study, and access to clinical paradigms that enhance the basic scientists' view of their biology. For example, the developmental biologist studying the role of RET oncogene mutations in neuronal signaling may know of its relationship to Hirschsprung's disease but may have limited insight into the clinical variability of Hirschsprung's disease. The biologist could thus fail to consider the panoply of other factors, networks, and epigenetic influences on this developmental program associated with enteric nervous system development.

Cultural awareness is a key component to effective career development for young physician-scientists, but too often this issue is not dealt with by either mentor or mentee. What do we mean by the "culture" of the academic medical center? Organizational structure and governance are of course important. Yet it is the informal ways in which faculty interact with one another, with administration, with trainees, and with the outside world that so greatly influence the day-to-day, minute-to-minute activities of the center. Each academic medical center has its own unique culture, which has generally evolved over many decades. Understanding the elements of this culture and its idiosyncrasies is essential for optimal career success in that environment. There are "cultures" that are very hierarchical ("top-down"). Others are silo-oriented. Some truly minimize barriers for junior faculty to gain access to the riches of the entire enterprise. One case in point: many highly motivated junior physician-scientists recognize that their ability to succeed academically is often related to access to critical state-of-the-art technology. This technology is frequently very expensive, and usually sits within the domain of a key faculty member or core center. Some academic centers optimize access to these types of enabling technology, while other centers make it practically impossible for new or junior faculty to gain access. To deal with the gatekeepers is often a challenge, the political nuances of which must be understood.

Conclusion

The relative decline in federal support for research has accompanied the decline in the physician-scientist population. The situation for the pediatric physician-scientist is even more striking. Between 1994 and 2005, although the NIH budget doubled under strong leadership, the pediatric portfolio fell from 14.1 percent to 11.3 percent of NIH funding (Gitterman et al. 2004). During FY1995–2001 success rates grew from 26.6 percent to 35.4 percent for internists but from 23.1 percent to 31 percent for pediatrics. Success rates in FY2001 for members of departments of neurology (34.9 percent) and psychiatry (32.3 percent) were stronger (Rangel et al. 2002).

Indeed, published reports in top-tier journals including *Science, Nature, Proceedings of the National Academy of Sciences USA, Journal of Clinical Investigation,* and the *New England Journal of Medicine* from American departments of pediatrics decreased by 35 percent from 2000 to 2006 (Rivkees and Genel 2007). Among the multitude of reasons is the high cost of developing pediatric physician-scientists. This is especially true for academic pediatric departments in which manpower for revenue generation is both currently limited (Jobe et al. 2002) and for which Medicaid, the predominant insurer (often exceeding 50 percent), provides extremely low reimbursement.

The perspective we have tried to convey in this chapter is that the development of a physician-scientist requires an evolutionary mentoring program. The needs of the trainees, whether medical student, resident, fellow, or junior faculty, differ at each stage of career development and provide a unique opportunity to focus on evolving academic and personal goals.

Formal mentoring should include both the dissemination of information (seminars, faculty guidelines) and periodic evaluation by the research mentor and departmental colleagues during the pre-faculty years. Formal involvement by the chair, section chief, and, most important, faculty development committees with broad oversight over the career progress of junior faculty from many sections is an essential component of career development and retention of junior faculty.

Protected time for research is key to a stable early career. It should be made clear to junior faculty members at the outset whether their start-up package covers only laboratory personnel for three years or five years or whether salary support for the junior faculty member is also included. Some young faculty are surprised to learn that, while salaries for their laboratory personnel may be covered during the start-up period, they themselves will be expected to do clinical work if they have not funded a certain percentage of their salary within the same timeframe.

Mentoring can also be provided informally by the opportunity to observe physician-scientists in action both in academia and in the home. Mentors frequently require training in how to give feedback, both positive and negative. Similarly, mentees often need coaching in how to accept constructive criticism. A shortage of role models in some areas (e.g., successful female physician-scientists in tenured faculty positions) may be addressed by multi-institutional mentoring grants such as the Pediatric Scientist Development Program, in which candidates with high potential are nominated at one institution but may train at another.

Clarity of expectation, transparent provision of financial support, and equity of access to other needed resources are the purview of the mentor and the institution. We contend that an approach to mentoring that is based on stage of career is one of the best ways to develop the physician-scientists who will populate our faculties for years to come.

On a personal note, academic pediatrics has been relatively spared a worrisome trend, that is, the formulaic and Relative Value Unit (RVU)–based clinical compensation models. This issue, however, now appears to be rapidly emerging in academic pediatrics as well. This is particularly challenging for the pediatric physician-scientist. The issue is complex. No two academic departments have identical compensation plans. That said, the recent movement toward clinical billing-allocated or time-allocated compensation models poses particular threats to the pediatric-scientist. Perhaps more than in any other medical specialty, the span of clinical specialization and clinical payments in pediatrics is wide ranging. In pediatrics there are very few "technical" specialties and far, far fewer patients in need of them than for comparable adult specialties (e.g., endoscopy, interventional cardiology, electrophysiology, bronchoscopy, organ transplantation). The pediatric specialty with both the largest patient volume and largest earning capacity is neonatology/newborn intensive care. The vast majority of pediatric specialists cannot "earn" their academic salaries (including the academic "overhead" costs), especially given the huge Medicaid burden and onerous Medicaid reimbursement schedule (generally much lower than with Medicare). This places the pediatric specialist in particular jeopardy, given pediatric academic center finances and current federal research funding trends.

Will our pediatric investigators of the near future be only neonatologists, cardiologists, or gastroenterologists? Where will the physician-scientists for pediatric genetics, rheumatology, infectious disease, diabetes, immunology, and nephrology be trained? Just as we have seen a dramatic shift in career choices of MSTP graduates in recent years (with markedly increased numbers and percentages electing "lifestyle specialties" such as dermatology, ophthalmology, and radiology over internal medicine, pediatrics, and pathology), pediatrics is at the threshold of a similar trend. The main drivers are likely to be income, lifestyle, and clinical billing–based protected time. The solutions are not simple. They involve philosophical issues; market forces; federal, state, and private payment systems; and institutional priorities and rewards to name but a few. Perhaps most important, a solution requires institutional leadership—leadership with both a passion for the development of pediatric physician-scientists and the determination to make difficult decisions to support them.

12

The Attrition of Young Physician-Scientists

PROBLEMS AND POTENTIAL SOLUTIONS

Mark Donowitz, MD, James Anderson, MD, PhD,
Fabio Cominelli, MD, PhD, and Greg Germino, MD

There is little doubt of the important and growing role played by the physician-scientist in generating medical advances in the post-genomic era.[1] Without extensive involvement of scientists who understand both basic physiologic mechanisms and the subtle aspects of human diseases, there will be significant delays in the application of molecular break-throughs to the diagnosis of diseases and the development of cures. With this in mind, the current situation of physician-scientists selecting investigative careers bears some scrutiny. As discussed in chapter 14 by Andrew Schafer, the Association of Professors of Medicine (APM) in its 2007 conference "Revitalizing the Nation's Physician-Scientist Work-force" (Nabel 2008; Ley 2005) concluded that we currently have fewer physician-scientists than are needed to take advantage of the opportunities to improve the health of our citizens. In order to illuminate the causes of and treatments for diseases, it is not only necessary to apply powerful new molecular, cell biologic, and genetic techniques so that we can better understand biologic processes but also essential to apply these advances directly to increase our understanding of how abnormalities in these processes produce human diseases.

Previous chapters have highlighted the fact that, despite the doubling of the National Institutes of Health (NIH) budget that ended in 2003, the

---

1. Parts of this chapter have been adapted from Donowitz et al. 2007.

total number of physician-scientists involved in NIH-sponsored research has not increased in over twenty-five years (approximately fifteen thousand). In contrast, the number of PhD scientists applying for NIH funding has increased continually during the same period (Ley and Rosenberg 2005; Nabel 2008; Ley 2005). For instance, the number of PhDs applying to the NIH for the first time has increased by almost 100 percent since the mid-1980s (Ley and Rosenberg 2005; Ley 2005), and in 2004 was approximately 2,800, compared to 1,200 MDs plus MD-PhDs (Dickler et al. 2007). This represents only a fraction of the total PhD pool currently competing for NIH funding.

As Timothy Ley has pointed out in chapter 2, simply to maintain the present physician-scientist workforce (not to increase it) will require an estimated five hundred to one thousand new physician-scientists per year, assuming the current rate of attrition remains constant. In a rapidly graying workforce, the average age of NIH principal investigators (PIs) is almost fifty-one and that of first-time NIH RO1 holders is over forty-two. The percent of PIs who are sixty-five to eighty years old increased from 0.8 percent in 1980 to 6.6 percent in 2006, with a projected rise to 11.2 percent by 2020 (Nabel 2008). This group of senior investigators will eventually stop being productive or will retire, bringing about the potential collapse of this vital research workforce.

Several streams feed the pool of physician-scientists. Each stream faces significant challenges. The major sources include the MD-PhD training programs and the so-called "late bloomer" MDs who gain their scientific training while in subspecialty fellowship programs. An estimated six hundred MD-PhD students graduate each year, who could theoretically provide the majority of the replacement pool. This is the medical training group that has the greatest chance of entering an investigative career. Although we do not know how their dropout rate compares to those of other groups of physician-scientists, we do know that many will not continue on the physician-scientist track.

On the one hand, of those physician-scientists entering MD-PhD programs, the number of men has remained about constant for fifteen years. On the other hand, the number of women has been increasing for the past decade, now constituting about 40 percent of the total. In spite of growing gender parity at entry, however, women have a higher attrition rate than their male colleagues as they try to ascend the faculty ladder (Ley and Rosenberg 2005; Nabel 2008; Ley 2005). The high attrition of women is a problem that must be solved in order to ensure the long-term stability of the workforce, as described by Reshma Jagsi and Nancy Tarbell in chapter 5. Not adequately considered as yet for their contribution to the physician-scientist pool are non-U.S.-trained physicians with strong scientific interests who receive research training in this country as a way of entering the American medical system. While this motivated group is likely to desire to contribute as physician-scientists, because of the need for clinical retraining, their age at entry will be a deterrent to some.

Of at least as much concern as the reluctance of physicians to undertake investigative careers is the significant dropout rate for those who have set out on this career path. Furthermore, there is no evidence that only the least capable physician-investigators drop out. Many of the potentially most creative physician-scientists abandon research careers. The result is that a huge personal and national investment in intellectual capital is being wasted.

The endangered status of physician-investigators has been an issue for over two decades. A number of interventions have been implemented to enhance the attractiveness of this career path—with variable success. Despite these well-intentioned efforts, the problem has not merely persisted but even worsened. In this chapter we analyze the magnitude of the attrition of physician-scientists and identify some of the reasons why young investigators abandon this career. We have identified a previously overlooked component of the career that we think is an important factor. More important, we enumerate some solutions that address this problem and might make this career path more attractive. At a time when other countries are expanding their investment in medical research and training, these solutions could also prevent the waste of American intellectual capital that we have identified.[2]

The Problems

One obvious deterrent to an investigative career is the large and increasing salary differential between physician-investigators and their peers who are full-time clinical practitioners. Nevertheless, this is probably more a disincentive to entry into the physician-scientist pathway than to continuing on it. Moreover, anecdotal evidence suggests that this differential is not the most important deterrent to physician-scientists deciding

---

2. The analysis presented takes liberally from data provided by Elizabeth Nabel, MD, director of the National Heart, Lung and Blood Institute (Nabel 2008), and Timothy Ley, MD, a contributor to this volume (Ley 2005). The problems identified and solutions suggested arose from a working group of the American Gastroenterological Association Institute Research Policy Committee (Drs. James Anderson, Fabio Cominelli, Alan Walker, Nick Davidson, Daniel Podolsky, and Kim Barrett) and several others (Drs. Mordecai Blaustein, Ann Hubbard, and Greg Germino).

to remain in an investigative career. There have always been physicians who are motivated by considerations beyond income, and the physician-scientist often fits this mold.

The combination of a lower salary and a perceived high risk of failure, however, may be a much more powerful consideration. In fact the reality as well as the perception for young scientists watching their more established role models attempt to continue in careers as physician-scientists is that most will fail. If one fears that he or she is more likely than not to fail, why take on the additional financial risks as well? The perception that one is likely to fail may also contribute to the high attrition rate of investigators already in the pipeline. Negative reviews of a submitted grant or paper may be viewed as a sign of things to come, triggering a decision to leave the career path prematurely. The investigator may decide, "Why delay the inevitable?" The higher the overall attrition rate, the more likely an individual may feel that he or she is also likely to fail, further increasing the attrition rate in a destructive positive-feedback loop.

Loan indebtedness is also frequently cited as an important factor. To counter this, in 2002 the NIH initiated a highly successful loan forgiveness program that is helping to lower barriers for interested trainees and may increase the number of candidates who enter the investigative pathway (Kotchen et al. 2004; Nathan 2002). This does not, however, address the dropout problem once investigators have already entered this pathway.

A Flawed Business Plan

Our analysis suggests that the lack of "business" security for individuals leading research laboratories is the issue of greatest concern for the physician-scientist. In addition to the intellectually creative aspects of science, running a successful research program presents all the challenges of running a small business and more. First, there is rent for laboratory space (paid by indirect costs on grants), as well as issues of managing personnel; compliance with health, safety, ethics, and animal and human studies standards; buying equipment; managing budgets; and finding funds to pay salaries for postdoctoral fellows and technicians. Support for this small business is most often sought by competing for NIH and foundation funds, which are increasingly difficult to obtain. What is even more challenging than for a small business is the fact that research programs are not-for-profit. They do not generate reserves and capital to carry them over during downturns. Indeed they are at risk of largely losing the ability to function if a single grant is turned down. Also, the amount of money provided from grants for the physician-scientist's salary is often insufficient

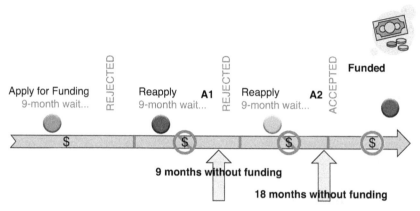

Figure 12.1. Funding process timeline for new RO1 funding. Figure was drawn in collaboration with Jessica Duncan and the American Gastroenterological Association.

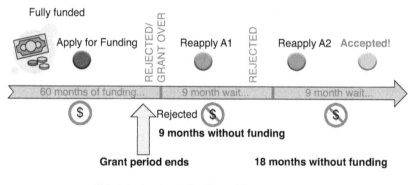

Figure 12.2. Flawed business plan of NIH-supported investigation.

to "purchase" the real percentage of effort required to accomplish the research. Clearly this is *not* a business model designed by an MBA.

The basic concept (see figures 12.1 and 12.2) is that the investigator's "small business" has a series of bills that come due predictably and continually. The ability to pay these bills comes in waves, however, with NIH funding achieved in a less predictable and often interrupted manner. It is these down periods which the investigator fears, since these are periods of "bankruptcy" for which the investigator has little ability to prepare by investing his or her income. Currently not more than 25 percent of the funds from any NIH grant can be carried over past the budget year, and the ability of an individual investigator to raise additional funds through philanthropy or by seeking investors in his or her research is very limited. These periods of bankruptcy, which often require laying off trained research personnel, also cause graduate students and postdoctoral fellows—individuals who in sum represent the intellectual capital of the laboratory—to rethink their projects.

Moving Toward a Solution

To assist in the development of appropriate solutions, we first identified the critical periods when physician-scientists are most likely to drop out of the investigator track. Typically, after successful completion of subspecialty training that includes a research fellowship component, the physician-scientist becomes a junior faculty member and applies for funding to support protected time for further training and development of an area of research. At this stage the five-year K series of mentored NIH training awards supports the research under the guidance of a mentor. NIH RO1 grants subsequently provide up to five years of independent support for each successful application. The data show that if physician-investigators are not able either to renew their first RO1 grant or to obtain a second RO1 grant, they are very likely to abandon the research track (Dickler et al. 2007; Kotchen et al. 2004).[3] The most vulnerable points for risk of attrition occur during the transition from K to RO1 funding, and in the attempt to renew the first RO1 grant or obtain a second RO1 grant, both of which are highly competitive processes.

We therefore scrutinized the available data regarding the outcomes for grant applications by physician-scientists (MD and MD-PhD) at each step in their early career pathway. Data were obtained from the NIH and the Association of American Medical Colleges (Dickler et al. 2007), and are also in part referred to in chapter 3 by David Korn and Stephen Heinig and chapter 2 by Timothy Ley. The success rate of physician-investigators in obtaining K awards has been, until recently, about 40 percent. Of the K award holders, about 80 percent applied for and about 60 percent received an

---

3. Data provided by W. T. Schaffer, PhD, NIH Senior Scientific Advisor for Extramural Research, and by Dr. D. Fang of the Association of American Medical Colleges.

R series grant, after up to three application attempts. The first-time success rate for individuals with MD or combined MD-PhD degrees who applied for R funding was 31 percent—higher for MD-PhDs (34 percent) than for MDs (28 percent). This demonstrates the importance of the K award program (Dickler et al. 2007). Of note, some physician-scientists who failed in obtaining their first RO1 grant applied for a different type of R grant (Dickler et al. 2007). Between 76 and 85 percent of first RO1 grant holders applied for competitive renewal of the grant or a second RO1 grant. Of these, approximately 73 percent (70 percent for MDs, 78 percent for MD-PhDs) were successful (Dickler et al. 2007). There are, however, no data indicating the percentage of physician-scientists who start this career pathway by applying for K support who are still involved at the later stages. If the stated rates of success for each career step (K, first RO1 grant, and its renewal) were all independent, then the probabilities of success at each stage could be multiplied to calculate the percentage of physician-scientists still applying for NIH funding when they finish competing for their second R award. This calculation provides a success rate of 11–12 percent for those physician-scientists starting on a K award–based pathway.

This level of success appears lower than what most of us have observed, indicating that success at one stage may not predict success at other stages. Research funding is also available from alternate sources such as the Department of Veterans Affairs, private foundations, and industry, providing some, though limited, additional opportunities to sustain investigative careers. Of course those who start this career path but no longer have research as their major activity may become leaders in other arenas of academic medicine that do not emphasize basic research. Nonetheless, despite potential flaws in the initial assumption that limit the accuracy of this estimate, these figures are still indicative of the difficulty of this career path. It also should be noted that the data cited are historical in nature and may not reflect the effects of the more recent flattening of the NIH budget.

Recommendations

Despite the high risks, many physicians continue to be attracted to research careers. By addressing some of the factors that lead to a high rate of attrition and thereby reducing the perceived high risk of such a career path, we will likely increase the number of trainees who enter this pathway. Beyond the flawed business model, many of the current policies of both the NIH and academic institutions may also be contributing to the high attrition. In addition to its well-received initiatives to reduce the burden of debt for those entering research careers, the NIH has considered ways to shorten the training process, including for physician-investigators. Because physician-scientists are already often insufficiently prepared to compete with PhDs for NIH funding, this must be thoughtfully deliberated.

One attempt by the NIH to increase the number of grants with a shorter duration of funding (RO3 and R21 grants offering only two to three years of support) is unlikely to be effective, given the enormous time commitment involved in applying for any R series grant. This initiative may increase rather than reduce the number of hurdles and lengthen the time before true stability is achieved. It actually threatens to increase the dropout rate of physician-scientists even further.

We therefore describe some alternative recommendations, including several that were considered at the APM conference "Revitalizing the Nation's Physician-Scientist Workforce." We also provide some recommendations that we think better address the underlying problem, adding some security for physician-scientists as they develop their "small businesses." These are particularly aimed at the two key transition times when attrition is highest. The solutions require commitments on the part of both the NIH and medical schools. Unquestionably the NIH has been aggressively committed to finding ways to address issues affecting the young investigator, particularly the young physician-scientist. We applaud these attempts. They demonstrate that solutions to this problem largely depend on changes within the institutions involved in developing the careers of physician-scientists. Although not all solutions will apply to each institution, the general principles do apply broadly. Local conditions must determine the best set of effective strategies for each medical school and academic medical center.

Recommended Changes Directed at the NIH

There are compelling reasons to recommend reinstitution of a specific award for first-time independent NIH applicants in the R series of awards, which are for five years and are funded at levels similar to grants for established investigators. This was also suggested in the 2005 National Research Council of the National Academies report titled "Bridge to Independence: Fostering the Independence of New Investigators in Biomedical Research" (National Research Council of the National Academies 2005). The concept of the old R29 (FIRST Award) was correct but provided too little funding to protect young investigators' research time and to allow them to develop scientifically.

The review process for these grants should discourage "triage." This is the current screening process that denies full peer review of grant applications which are initially considered to rank in the bottom half of submissions in any given review cycle. It creates the very harmful effect of telling first-time applicants that their work is not even good enough to merit the time and effort of the reviewers, thereby depriving them of the helpful input that discussion of applications often provides. The criteria for review of these applications should focus more on the importance of the question asked. They should not expect extensive amounts of preliminary data but rather should consider the scientific expertise of the candidate gained through training. Of note is the policy in some NIH institutes of funding first-time investigators who receive lower priority scores than established investigators ("handicapping"). While this will allow first-time funding to increase, it may not encourage staying in beyond the initial grant. This preferable funding of first-time applicants is likely to create two pools of investigators—one young and one old—with the potentially most pro-ductive group (mature but not yet old investigators) falling through the cracks.

The NIH's K099 grant, also called the K/R award, may prove to be an important funding mechanism. This is a five-year award that involves a mentored component (first two years) followed by three years of independent investigator-initiated funding that can be transferred to any institution at which the candidate obtains an independent faculty position. The award has the potential to shorten the training period for physician-investigators while allowing them to continue working with their mentors, since the transition to independence must be proposed in a coordinated manner (Nabel 2008). This could indeed reduce the problem of the advanced age of first-time NIH PIs. At this writing only a relatively small number of such awards had been made, primarily to PhDs. NIH leadership has, however, recognized the potential importance of this award and is considering increasing the number and opening it to physician-scientists. There is also laudable consideration of making it a seven-year award by expanding the independent component to five years. Furthermore, suggestions of increasing support for all K awards and expanding the period of funding to seven years is consistent with the longer time it takes to initiate independent research careers and the need to purchase time for the K awardee to do the science.

It will also be important to provide increased security by making an additional amount of money available for K awardees who are clearly attempting to achieve R funding and for initial RO1 holders attempting either to renew their first RO1 or to obtain a second RO1 grant. This could be built in as anticipated carryover (perhaps called "guaranteed bridge support") and awarded if the applicant is unsuccessful in obtaining continuous funding. An additional requirement could mandate review at the academic institution that documents continued commitment to an investigative career. This additional funding should be sufficient for maintenance of research infrastructure and not used for faculty salaries.

There is an urgent need for analysis of the amount of support required to maintain the physician-scientist pool. The NIH Office for Portfolio Analysis and Strategic Initiatives should analyze data on early career development, recommend an "ideal" level of support required to sustain the pipeline of physician-scientist investigators for the next generation, and use this information to recommend additional initiatives aimed at recruiting and retaining the MD investigator.

Recommended Changes Directed at Academic Institutions

There are serious concerns that academic institutions have not sufficiently committed themselves or their resources to the development and maintenance of the physician-scientist workforce. Rather medical schools have been too often satisfied with providing the framework for this career development without adequate consideration of what it takes today to achieve success for the individual physician-scientist and consequently for the larger scientific enterprise. This said, there are exemplary exceptions, which at an individual institutional level have paid a great deal of attention to developing, maintaining, and enhancing the careers of their physician-scientists.

Given limited resources, it will be important to increase institutional involvement in the intramural selection of which physician-scientists to develop, as well as in the process of their development. More critical institutional oversight is needed in identifying candidates who have the qualifications and the durable commitment to enter the physician-scientist pathway. Oversight would also include monitoring progress during the initial years of career development. Most institutions seem to follow a laissez-faire approach to deciding which physician-scientists should attempt to develop an academic career, which generally means competing for NIH career awards as a first step. The APM conference distinguished between the two major approaches used for physician-scientist career development as "the guppy method" and the "prolonged investment method." In the former, many candidates start out but few are successful, with their institutions investing little capital in their career development beyond an initial "package." Even these initial start-up funds are often too limited for internally hired trainees, who are immediately placed at a competitive disadvantage compared to new faculty members recruited from the outside. They are often vastly undercapitalized, and thus put at very high risk of failure. In the latter model, the institution typically hires far fewer young faculty but then expects to invest in their careers at multiple points in their career development.

The difference in these methods can be emphasized by describing examples of each. In the former, if a mentor encourages a candidate to pursue a physician-scientist career, the mentor and young physician-scientist develop a career pathway with relatively little investment from the institution. The career plan typically involves application for NIH K award funding, often with success in the application being a condition for receiving a faculty appointment. Office, laboratory space, and start-up funds are negotiated on an individual basis. Many of the most successful physician-scientists in our current system have come via this pathway. Nevertheless, many of those who embark on this path find that teaching or clinical activities fit their career goals better than research and use the K awards to develop these aspects of their careers, becoming important clinician-educators over time. The successes of K awardees who have developed their careers by this mechanism are used to justify the approach. Even if this group is highly successful, the institutions are not adequately committed to providing support later in their careers when they hit the expected bumps in the road of NIH funding. The prolonged investment model does not represent a "welfare state" for investigators. When funding lapses occur, the careers of the physician-scientists are critically analyzed at the medical school level for quality and quantity of work as well as the potential for future contributions. After repeated assessment, further investments in the career are made so that the "small business" is not closed.

We suggest that academic medical centers should cultivate new methods for the institutional development of physician-scientist careers, both to reduce the early turnover and to improve the return on the NIH investment. Institutions that want to participate in competing for NIH K award funding should be required to organize institutional K awardee evaluation committees. Such committees would interview the prospective K award applicant and his or her mentor to understand the quality of the research career proposed. These committees would also assess the motivation of both applicant and mentor in seeking the award, and determine whether or not the application—and, more important, the investigative career of the applicant—has a reasonable chance of long-term success.

This committee would then meet on a regular basis with the K awardee and mentor to determine whether the investigative career development warrants continued NIH support, evaluate the mentoring system in place, and help determine when it is appropriate for the K awardee to apply for R funding. This would give the institution the responsibility of helping to assess the career development of the physician-scientist, which is now increasingly recognized as involving multiple components. These include different aspects of mentoring, further education, and a large percent of protected time. Conversely, the committee might determine when it is clear that a K awardee has decided that the career he or she wishes to pursue is not primarily in research. The committee would then be charged with working with the K awardee, mentor, and institution to return the balance of the K award to the NIH, since these awards are intended exclusively to increase the research mission of institutions.

As part of the monitoring of the young physician-scientist, the rules for time commitment of a K awardee need to be more carefully defined. It is suggested that 80 percent research commitment, which is required of K awardees, be based on a forty-hour workweek, and consequently only eight hours per week should be available for non-research activities (clinical service, teaching, committee participation). Monitoring this time distribution would be part of the committee's responsibility. This approach is likely to free up some NIH funds which could be recycled. This is critical because the number of K awards (or K/R awards) cannot support the five hundred to one thousand physicians who must enter the system annually to maintain the current steady-state number of physician-scientists.

For holders of a first R series award, the mentor should be required to organize a faculty committee that would meet at least annually to provide a written report to the NIH describing progress, time spent in research, and the potential for and continued interest in research. Analysis of time spent in non-investigative activities should be provided, including time in educational, clinical, and administrative functions.

Formal mentoring should be arranged and its effectiveness monitored. This is important for all young physician-scientists but has been given particularly insufficient attention for issues more common in the careers of women and underrepresented minorities. The need for multiple mentors is particularly important for women, as they can face challenges not only in scientific direction but also in determining how to integrate an investigative career into family issues including child rearing responsibility. These mentoring considerations are more fully developed in other chapters.

As described further elsewhere in this book, institutions need to accept more directly the challenge to expand the number of women physician-scientists. Increasingly candidates for the physician-scientist workforce come from the pool of women who are entering this career path but dropping out early in numbers that exceed the male attrition rate. Today we find that male partners increasingly share—or even shoulder—child care responsibilities. Nonetheless, bringing up families generally remains more an area of responsibility for women. Institutions should therefore continue the trend of innovating ways to allow women to have investigative careers while taking part in bringing up their families. Notably, the concept has been proposed that physician-scientists play different roles in research groups based on the stage of their careers. For instance, a physician-scientist could be a co-investigator but not a PI during the early years of a career and only later become a PI, with the added responsibilities required.

Academic institutions have to a large extent taken part in physician-scientist career development at the entry level by providing space and start-up packages for their new recruits. But recall that the "business model" in which NIH grant funding is intermittent, taking several rounds of applications for even the best investigators with the best applications. Given this fact, institutions should develop systems that routinely provide bridge funding for the investigators they wish to retain.

We suggest that medical schools develop committees that they charge to use criteria of past accomplishments and future promise to decide which of their physician-scientists they want to retain by supporting them during the period in which they attempt to achieve NIH funding. Each academic medical center is likely to have somewhat different goals and local politics; but this form of institutional investment to support the NIH investment would contribute significantly to reversing the problem of attrition. Indeed it is surprising that the NIH has not insisted that its investments in physician-scientists be complemented more comprehensively at the institutional level. This proposal has the potential to increase the security of physician-scientists in maintaining their critical laboratory personnel. Our analysis suggests that this lack of security—the ever present concern that with every NIH application it is possible that laboratory personnel will have to be let go—is a major reason why physician-scientists abandon investigative careers.

In response to the likely institutional lament that they lack the funds to provide bridging or continued investment in their physician-scientists, we note the increasing endowments of many academic medical centers, although the economic downturn must be considered over the short-term. Raising endowments for bridging appears to be achievable for all research-intensive institutions, especially if this is made a requirement for institutional eligibility to submit K or R award applications. Furthermore, to some extent the expenses saved from becoming more selective in initial investment in starting up investigators could be redirected to consolidating support for highly productive investigators already in the system.

Institutions offer potentially important academic benefits that can help those physician-scientists who take advantage of them. Sabbaticals are such a benefit. It is suggested that institutions develop methods for increasing the transparency of the resources they make available for such benefits. For instance, including education about the advantages of taking a sabbatical and how sabbaticals can be pursued most productively should be part of the mentoring of new faculty.

The plight of young physician-scientists has rightly caught the attention of many thought leaders in the community. Some proposed solutions for how institutions can support physician-scientists do not seem helpful. For example, a suggestion that institutions pay salaries for established senior investigators to free up NIH money for young investigators seems to have the potential for misuse. Peer review now determines when senior scientists are no longer able to maintain their laboratories. Guaranteeing their time at the institutional level might prolong research careers that are no longer competitive. The money is probably better used for providing bridge funding for those who continue to do cutting-edge research.

Physician-scientists can choose to pursue basic or clinical research, and we have not separated out the outcomes for each pathway, nor do we find it productive to focus on only one path. The basic challenges are nevertheless very similar, and we feel that the changes we have outlined should be pursued as a requirement to ensure the viability of both.

How Much Money Should be Invested in the Young Physician-Scientist?

In considering the plight of the physician-scientist, two items particularly stand out as needing urgent attention. First, given the limited money available for physician-scientist career development, we need a national debate on how we are to distribute these funds between young investigators, who represent future promise, and established investigators, who are currently conducting groundbreaking and clinically promising studies. There is no clearly articulated strategy on how the funds are to be distributed, and this is hindering decisions on how much to invest in the young investigator. This question needs to be discussed in the context of our true manpower needs. The frequent attention given to this problem suggests that current levels are inadequate. Nonetheless, formal analysis is needed to enable informed decisions regarding how to balance competing needs and interests with economic realities. If objective studies truly predict a serious shortage, we may have to implement bolder strategies aimed at both recruitment and retention.

Second, for over twenty years the academic medical community has repeatedly expressed concern about the fate of the physician-investigator and then responded with a series of interventions. Regrettably it seems that these policies and actions have failed to provide substantive solutions. One important reason for our repeated failure to solve the problem may be that we have not yet adequately defined all of its root causes. Solutions have been drawn up for problems identified on a very incomplete dataset. In this chapter we have identified another reason why prior strategies have been unsuccessful and proposed interventions that we think will at least partially address those shortcomings. But even our observations are more anecdotal than evidence based. We urgently need improved tools to track the course of our young physician-investigators and to identify the reasons why those who drop out choose to do so.

Conclusions

Fostering investigative careers for physicians is in the best interest of the developed world, which cannot afford to continue to waste so much intellectual capital. We have identified an important reason that accounts for much of this wasted investment in the United States, and we have suggested changes that should make this career pathway more attractive. The lack of comprehensive data on this topic warrants a national effort to define it better. A broad discussion involving multiple constituencies is required to guide future investment strategies that balance the needs of new versus established investigators (Zerhouni 2005). Finally, it is recommended that this discussion include the broader question of the role of physician-scientists in the biomedical enterprise, the overarching topic of this book. We must understand the projected number required for the success of physician-scientists as meaningful contributors to medical research, as well as the relative roles of the NIH and academic institutions in securing their future. Together these data can be used to devise the most effective strategies for continuing to push back the frontiers of understanding, preventing, and treating human disease.

13

Restoring and Invigorating an "Endangered Species"

INITIATIVES BY THE ASSOCIATION OF AMERICAN MEDICAL COLLEGES

David Korn, MD, and Stephen J. Heinig

In this chapter we review lessons from a national "clinical research summit" meeting that embedded academic clinical research within the larger construct of a national clinical research enterprise, and from the Association of American Medical Colleges' (AAMC) initial task force on clinical research that recommended wide-ranging organizational and programmatic reforms to strengthen clinical investigation in medical schools, teaching hospitals, and health care systems. We then discuss the recommendations of a second AAMC task force on clinical research, which focused exclusively on concrete and measurable actions to strengthen the environment for academic clinical and translational physician-scientists. We conclude by summarizing the concomitantly sustained efforts by the AAMC and the academic community to strengthen the integrity of clinical investigation in the face of mounting government, media, and public concerns about academic medicine's steadily deepening interactions with industry.

A Call to Action

The AAMC's first initiative in support of clinical research was the National Clinical Research Summit Project, in concert with the Wake Forest University School of Medicine and the American Medical Association (AMA). The idea of a summit was proposed in 1997 by Thompson and Moskowitz (both then at Wake Forest) in a *JAMA* editorial (Thompson and

Moskowitz 1997) occasioned by reports of the adverse impact of managed care and cost containment on clinical research (Campbell, Weissman, and Blumenthal 1997).

The objective of the Clinical Research Summit, chaired by William Danforth, chancellor emeritus of Washington University in St. Louis, was to develop a base of commitment and support for clinical research, broadly defined, across all sectors of society that contribute to and benefit from such research. In a process designed to distill the most salient observations and, where possible, consensus from its many diverse participants, ten focus groups were established comprising more than 150 representatives of government and private-sector funding agencies, the biotechnology and pharmaceutical industries, corporate and government purchasers of health care, health plans and insurance companies, patient advocates, ethicists, leaders and representatives of academic medical centers, junior and senior medical research faculty, and others. In November 1998 representatives from all focus groups convened for the "summit meeting" in Winston-Salem, North Carolina, to synthesize their work products into a coherent and comprehensive set of objectives and recommendations. The final report embraced a broad definition of clinical research (see text box 13.1) and articulated the vision of a structure to promote a balanced agenda of clinical research; the structure was dubbed the "national clinical research enterprise" (Association of American Medical Colleges and the American Medical Association 1998). The summit meeting generated an expansive and inclusive vision of "clinical research" that extended from the earliest steps of translation of basic science findings into human health and disease to the ultimate adoption of new insights into evidence-based clinical practice.

The focus groups profoundly challenged the AAMC's member organizations with the failure, despite decades of introspection and proclaimed parochial concerns, to establish an empirical or objectively demonstrable case for a shared *national* emergency with respect to the state of academic clinical investigation. Especially critical were business representatives to the summit, some whose own industries had undergone jarring economic dislocations with no ensuing claims of national urgency or pleas for federal relief. The nonacademics, while sympathetic to the difficulties faced by new physician-scientists and other investigators, were decidedly unsympathetic to what they perceived as academic "whining." This external perspective was invaluable in motivating the AAMC to undertake further analyses and in framing its public advocacy on behalf of clinical and translational research.

The summit concluded that there is in fact a shortage of adequately trained and supported clinical investigators in the United States, primarily in relation to the tremendous opportunities that have been made available

---

Text Box 13.1. Definition of Clinical Research from the Clinical Research Summit Project

Clinical research is a component of medical and health research intended to produce knowledge valuable for understanding disease, preventing and treating illness, and promoting health. Clinical research embraces a continuum of studies involving interaction with patients, diagnostic clinical materials or data, or populations in any of these categories.

• Disease mechanisms
• Translational research
• Clinical knowledge, detection, diagnosis, and natural history of disease
• Therapeutic interventions, including clinical trials
• Prevention and health promotion
• Behavioral research
• Health services research
• Epidemiology
• Community-based and managed care–based research (AAMC 2000)

Note: The AAMC's Clinical Research Task Force II used a modified definition of clinical research that focused primarily on the "first translational block."

---

through advancements in biomedical and behavioral research. This shortage, and the lack of enabling infrastructure, was particularly acute for new and emerging fields, such as health services research. Put succinctly, the summit saw the "crisis" in clinical research as one of lost opportunities and outsized public health needs. To help communicate to society the critically important role played by clinical research, an effective metaphor was devised: "Clinical research is the 'neck of the scientific bottle,' through which all scientific developments in biomedicine must flow before they can be of *real-world* benefit to the public" (Association of American Medical Colleges and the American Medical Association 1999, emphasis added). The intuitive understanding of clinical research as a bottleneck resonated with the public and members of Congress when the final report of the summit project (*A National Call to Action*) was released on Capitol Hill in December 1999.

The conferees underscored the lack of data appropriate to monitor and assess performance of the various components of clinical research and argued that the research system must move beyond measurement by financial inputs (e.g., funding and number of NIH grants):

> Ultimately, quantitative methods and evaluative methodologies should be developed to support analyses of clinical research productivity based upon diffusion of results into, and effects on, health care practice, the implementation of new strategies of disease therapy and prevention and health promotion, the development of new drugs, devices and medical procedures, and improvement in measures of population health status. (Association of American Medical Colleges and the American Medical Association 1999)

The summit proposed dedicating part of the Public Health Service's "1 percent evaluation tap" (on Department of Health and Human Services appropriations) for this purpose. Like the 1997 NIH Nathan panel (see chapter 3), the Clinical Research Summit Project also made suggestions for strengthening General Clinical Research Centers (GCRCs) and for a stronger emphasis on training programs in the ethical underpinnings of clinical research.

A final recommendation, intended to maintain the momentum generated by the summit initiative, led to the establishment by the Institute of Medicine (IOM) in 2000 of the Clinical Research Roundtable (Sung et al. 2003), which functioned until 2004, when it was disbanded and succeeded by such new IOM initiatives as the Evidence Based Medicine Roundtable and the Forum on Drug Discovery, Development, and Translation. Influenced by the summit, the AAMC's legislative agenda in 2000 included, for the first time, the association's support for the congressional Clinical Research Enhancement Act (CREA), championed by the American Federation for Medical Research and other Washington-based advocates, which expanded the scope of GCRCs, authorized creation of loan repayment programs for clinical and specified other biomedical investigators, and called for regular periodic evaluation of NIH clinical research programs, among other provisions. The CREA's provisions were incorporated into other legislation and signed into law that year (Food and Drug Administration 2000).

Task Force I

> The central challenge for medical schools and teaching hospitals is to attract the capital and human resources required for realizing the new era of clinical research, when fiscal constraints on the health delivery system from managed care and changes to federal Medicare and Medicaid programs

have transformed the original model of support. (AAMC Clinical Research
Task Force I, Association of American Medical Colleges 2000a)

The AAMC's first Task Force on Clinical Research (1998–2000), known
as CRTF I, worked in parallel with the Clinical Research Summit Project;
but in contrast to the summit, which focused on the environment for clinical research external to academic medical centers, the task force focused
on advising what the association and its member medical schools and
teaching hospitals should do themselves to strengthen clinical research
and training. CRTF I also saw itself as a complement to the NIH Nathan
panel, focusing on the institutions that perform most of the NIH-funded
clinical research and research training. "NIH funding by itself," the task
force observed, "will [never] be sufficient to undergird the future of clinical research in medical schools and teaching hospitals" (Association of
American Medical Colleges 2000a).

CRTF I developed recommendations for strengthening the organization and management of academic clinical research in four separate areas,
each of which is summarized later in this chapter: (1) training and career
development, (2) infrastructure, (3) integration of clinical research with
extended delivery systems, and (4) clinical trials. The task force used the
Summit Project's definition of clinical research and conducted surveys, site
visits, and case studies, as well as examining AAMC and NIH records.

CRTF I reminded academic medical centers of their strengths, declaring
that clinical research is a defining characteristic of medical schools and
teaching hospitals. These institutions are central to innovation in health
care because of their unique combination of assets and infrastructure,
including:

- An affiliated health care system
- Access to a large and diverse sample of patients motivated to partici-
  pate in clinical research
- A cadre of experienced clinical investigators across specialties and
  subspecialties
- Funding to support career development and faculty time for research
- Areas of basic science research excellence
- Niche areas of clinical excellence
- Access to philanthropy
- Opportunities for joint ventures with industry
- Opportunities to collaborate in research and teaching with affiliated
  public health schools and other units in the parent university, and
  other proximal academic institutions, health care delivery systems,
  and/or health maintenance organizations (HMOs)

- Training and education programs
- Presence of dedicated clinical research and service units (Association of American Medical Colleges 2000a)

With respect to education and training, CRTF I found that most medical students and residents were not being systematically exposed to high-quality clinical research, or clinical research models and mentors, as part of their professional development. Residency training requirements, as defined by the major accreditation and certification bodies, the Accreditation Council for Graduate Medical Education (ACGME) and the American Board of Medical Specialties (ABMS), varied widely in terms of required or permitted exposure to research during the training sequence. In spite of research requirements in some residencies and fellowships, few residents or clinical fellows actually received formal training in the tools and methods needed for conducting high-quality clinical research, and the training experiences themselves varied widely in length, intensity, and quality. While NIH training programs, including the career development programs created in response to the Nathan panel, were welcome, most of these programs did not cover significant institutional costs related to clinical research training.[1]

The task force also found an array of new programs in medical schools relevant to the education of clinical researchers but questioned the effectiveness of many and especially noted the lack of systematic curricula. CRTF reached no consensus on the optimal duration of such programs or the desirability of pursuing additional degrees at the master's or PhD level. In consideration of these points, CRTF I argued that it was incumbent on medical schools "to develop a culture supportive of clinical research and transmit the excitement of clinical research to medical students, residents and fellows" (Association of American Medical Colleges 2000a). CRTF I recommended that clinical research training programs must define a rigorous set of competencies, skills, and knowledge-based requirements for their program graduates. It further recommended promoting diversity and planning for long-term (multiyear) funding of trainees and a stable, long-term funding base for the program, and it declared that systematic outcomes data on early career choices and opportunities must be collected and analyzed to evaluate the efficacy of the new generation of clinical research training programs.

---

1. The task force noted in particular the Robert Wood Johnson Clinical Scholars Program as demonstrating the valuable role that health-related foundations can play in funding clinical research training.

With respect to clinical research infrastructure, CRTF I noted that traditionally, major responsibility for clinical research had been departmental, while emerging opportunities and required infrastructure for clinical
research increasingly involve multiple departments within the medical
school, teaching hospital, and other components of the university, as
well as linkages to other institutions (Mallon and Bunton 2005). Even the
GCRCs, which exemplified a coordinated effort to provide dedicated resources within the hospital setting to support largely inpatient clinical
research, were still far too limited in the task force's view. CRTF I called
for extending the mission of the GCRC to encompass the broader health
system, including outpatient services and settings beyond the campus.

While recognizing a number of new technologies with promise for research, CRTF I was perhaps most disappointed with the state of clinical
information systems in support of research.

While many medical schools and teaching hospitals have invested large
sums of money in clinical, administrative, and financial information systems, most have not invested in the enhancements that are necessary to
facilitate application to clinical research. Health services research has been
traditionally underemphasized. This represents a significant opportunity
for medical schools and teaching hospitals to enhance health care in their
local communities and strengthen their value to patients and the funders
of health care (Association of American Medical Colleges 2000a).

As a result of the CRTF I recommendations, the AAMC convened a
conference on October 30–31, 2002, supported by the National Science
Foundation, to consider approaches and policies to ensure that research
needs are incorporated within the design of clinical record-keeping and
information systems (Association of American Medical Colleges 2002a).
The conference recommended that NIH and other federal sponsors attend
more to standard-setting than to software and product development. The
standards, if successful, would be emulated by research organizations and
would provide incentives for vendors and firms to tailor their software
and systems accordingly. Now, over a decade since the CRTF I recommendations, we note sadly that many of these same issues—including issues
of standards and "interoperability of systems"—remain to be settled, despite attention from numerous, highly publicized national initiatives to
promote the adoption of electronic health records.

CRTF I noted continuing difficulties in the integration of clinical research
within the large extended academic delivery systems that were developing at the time. Many of these systems integrated, or would attempt to integrate, the services of one or several hospitals with a network of clinics
and other health providers in the effort to provide better and more efficient

health care to larger numbers of patients and subscribers while generating increased revenues for the academic medical center. At the same time, many universities and medical schools were divesting themselves of ownership in their affiliated hospitals and health systems. The task force found that, with few exceptions, clinical research was not integrated within the extended delivery systems evolving at many medical schools and teaching hospitals and that administrative responsibility for clinical research remained largely fragmented. "Most of the leaders in academic medicine view this situation as an opportunity lost" (Association of American Medical Colleges 2000a).

CRTF I cited as the best example of the systematic integration of research with delivery of care the National Cancer Institute's Comprehensive Cancer Centers. The task force noted two factors as critical to the centers' success: sufficient funding by NCI to offset the medical school's or teaching hospital's investments in infrastructure and administrative costs for the program; and the prestige, recognition, and increased patient volume that the affiliated delivery system accrued from being associated with excellence in cancer research and care. This citation seems prescient in light of the ambitious Clinical and Translational Science Awards (CTSA) program launched by NIH several years later. The CTSAs are intended to integrate disparate components from across campuses, health systems, and communities into a single organizational structure to facilitate and support clinical and translational research and training.

Clinical Trials Organization

CRTF I also examined the organization and administration of clinical trials in academic medical centers, which at the time was an issue of much concern given that the share of industry-sponsored clinical trials performed by medical schools and teaching hospitals had declined from 80 percent to 40 percent (Association of American Medical Colleges 2000a). The 1990s saw the rise of private contract research organizations (CROs), which serve as intermediaries between medical products industry sponsors and investigators at clinical trials sites, sometimes collaborating but more often competing with academic institutions depending on the specifics of each trial contract.

At the time of the CRTF I study, medical schools and teaching hospitals were pursuing varied strategies for managing industry-sponsored trials. The task force identified six models:

- An academic CRO-type organization
- A centralized clinical trials office

- A hybrid clinical trials office
- Traditional department- or investigator-based model of clinical trials
- Joint venture with an external CRO or site management organization
- Utilization of the services of an umbrella organization (Association of American Medical Colleges 2000a)

Although CRTF I determined that it had no evidence from which to recommend a particular model for all medical schools and teaching hospitals, it made several recommendations for better planning and evaluation of an institution's clinical trials operations. The AAMC, building on the CRTF's recommendations, compiled sample provisions from key areas of contention in negotiating clinical trials contracts (intellectual property, publication, indemnification, and medical care in case of adverse consequences) (Baer et al. 2004), but was unsuccessful in attempting jointly with the Pharmaceutical Research and Manufacturers of America to reach a consensus on "best language" between senior representatives of academic medicine and the pharmaceutical industry.

One of the arguments for more centralized management of clinical trials was to permit the institution to resist industry pressure to control critical aspects of clinical trial design and analysis, investigators' access to the primary data, and publication of results. Well after CRTF I adjourned, the AAMC, working with leading academic clinical trialists, ethicists, and medical journal editors, promulgated its "Principles for Protecting Integrity in the Conduct and Reporting of Clinical Trials" (Ehringhaus and Korn 2006). Sadly, only a single medical school (the University of Alabama at Birmingham) formally adopted the principles. Many school leaders expressed fear of disadvantaging their faculties in competing for industry-sponsored clinical trials, while noting that they supported the principles and would be prepared to adopt them if all the schools agreed to do so. As it happened, some of the key principles became instantiated by fiat of the International Committee of Medical Journal Editors (ICMJE) (De Angelis et al. 2004; also De Angelis et al. 2005), by the gratifying success of the National Library of Medicine's (NLM) clinical trials registry (accessible at clinicaltrials.gov), and by provisions in the FDA Authorization Act of 2007 (Food and Drug Administration 2007). The latter expanded the scope of the clinical trials registration mandate as well as the number of data elements that must be registered. It also required for the first time the reporting at clinicaltrials.gov of clinical trials results in a structured template that was developed by NLM and activated in October 2008.

Task Force II

> Academic medicine [must] produce and support sufficient cadres of trans-
> lational and clinical physician-scientists to propel scientific advances into
> better diagnostics, treatments, and preventatives of disease. Yet, concerns
> are widespread that organizational and cultural barriers in academic med-
> ical institutions are preventing this from happening. (CRTF II, Association
> of American Medical Colleges 2006b; Dickler, Korn, and Gabbe 2006)

Five years after CRTF I, the association conducted a series of surveys
of GCRC directors and research deans at medical schools and teaching
hospitals to determine the institutional changes aimed at facilitating clinical research that had taken place since the release of the CRTF I report.
While there had been some increase in new training programs (mostly
in response to the NIH K30 curriculum development awards) and other
improvements, many areas that CRTF I had identified as needing urgent
attention saw only marginal progress. For example, only six institutions
had a centralized structure supporting all or almost all aspects of clinical
research, although many more reported that they were planning to establish such structures (Association of American Medical Colleges 2006b;
Dickler, Korn, and Gabbe 2006).

The NIH funding environment for academic medical centers had also
changed in the intervening years. The NIH budget had doubled to $27.6 bil-
lion in 2003, and the Office of Management and Budget had indicated
that it planned no further real growth in the agency's funding for the remainder of the Bush administration, which was otherwise preoccupied
in any event. NIH director Elias Zerhouni had implemented a strategic
plan (the "NIH Roadmap") that included specific initiatives aimed at "reengineering the clinical research enterprise," leading to creation of new
career development awards (the Roadmap K12 and T32 awards) and later
the CTSA. Several years after implementation of the Nathan panel recommendations and the doubling of NIH funding, and during the ongoing
Roadmap process, new questions emerged regarding clinician-scientists'
success in competing for and completing the new NIH career development awards. What percentage of initial recipients of the new career development awards are on track to careers as independent investigators?
Was a new national initiative needed to stimulate structural change in
medical schools and teaching hospitals? Answering the last question in
the affirmative, AAMC convened its second Task Force on Clinical Research (CRTF II) in February 2005.

Like its predecessor, CRTF II had a broad charge that included matters of institutional infrastructure, but in executing the charge, CRTF II

became increasingly focused on the training and career development of clinical investigators. (Note that seven of the twelve recommendations in text box 13.2 are focused on training and career development.) In its work, CRTF II also limited itself to addressing only the so-called "first translational gap" as articulated by the IOM Clinical Research Roundtable (Sung et al. 2003), focusing exclusively on the recruitment, training, and sustenance of physician-scientists who play a key role in the "conception, design, and performance of hypothesis-driven, patient-oriented studies that are generally peer-reviewed and are commonly, but not exclusively, conducted in medical schools and teaching clinics and hospitals." In addition to making recommendations on training and career development, CRTF II also called for needed improvements to infrastructure (four recommendations) and finance (one recommendation, and that more of a plea) (Association of American Medical Colleges 2006b; Dickler, Korn, and Gabbe 2006).

Text Box 13.2. Recommendations of the AAMC Clinical Research Task Force II

1. Every future physician should receive a thorough education in the basic principles of clinical and translational research, both in medical school and during residency training.
2. The Liaison Committee on Medical Education (LCME) should add education in translational and clinical research to the requirements for medical school accreditation, and the Accreditation Council for Graduate Medical Education (ACGME) should embed understanding of translational and clinical research within its required core competencies.
3. Training for translational and clinical investigators should comprise completion of an advanced degree with a thesis project (or an equivalent educational experience), tutelage by an appropriate mentor, and a substantive postdoctoral training experience.
4. Sufficient support should be given to new junior faculty who are translational and clinical investigators to maximize their probability of success.
5. Training in translational and clinical research should be accelerated through comprehensive restructuring so that translational and clinical scientists can become independent clinicians and investigators at the earliest possible time.

6. Institutions, journals, the NIH, and other research sponsors should take steps to facilitate appropriate academic recognition of translational and clinical scientists for their contributions to collaborative research.
7. The NIH should modify the K23 and K24 awards to enhance their value in supporting clinical and translational research training and mentoring.
8. Institutions should provide central oversight, administration, and support for the essential infrastructure required by the translational and clinical research enterprise.
9. Human research protection programs (HRPPs) should be made more effective and efficient by (a) trans-agency harmonization of federal regulations, (b) accreditation of HRPPs, (c) simplification of institutional regulatory compliance processes, and (d) expanded use of central Institutional Review Boards in multi-site research.
10. A national forum should be established (a) to facilitate development of clinical information systems that integrate data from diverse clinical and research information platforms, and (b) to develop DNA and tissue banks that correlate genotypic and phenotypic data and ensure regulatory compliance.
11. Academic medical institutions should establish collaborations with community healthcare providers and practice-based research networks to broaden the diversity and size of the population base for translational and clinical research and to increase opportunities for health services, epidemiological, and outcomes research.
12. Medical schools and their affiliated teaching hospitals should explicitly recognize and vigorously promote translational and clinical research as a core mission and accord it a high priority for institutional funding.

Despite the proliferation of training and career development programs that represented a substantial commitment from the NIH and academic medical centers, these programs continued to vary widely in requirements and quality. As a consequence, the graduates of such programs could not consistently compete well with PhD and postdoctorate graduates in convincing department chairs and medical school deans of their likelihood of success in establishing themselves in sponsored research, and thus persuading them to commit the substantial institutional support necessary for establishing a new investigator. CRTF II presumed that if the quality of clinical research training was more consistent and rigorous, institutions would be more willing to support these newly hired faculty investigators with start-up packages and other resources comparable to those offered to basic sciences appointees. Thus the first three CRTF II recommendations echo and strengthen earlier recommendations of CRTF I. With respect to clinician-scientist training programs, CRTF II went beyond its predecessor in recommending that effective clinical research training should include a degree program (at minimum, at the master's level) with a core curriculum and a mentored thesis project, and that an additional period of two-to-three years of "rigorous, mentored 'postdoctoral' experience in clinical and translational research is necessary to prepare trainees for independence" (Association of American Medical Colleges 2006b; Dickler, Korn, and Gabbe 2006).

CRTF II's concerns, however, went beyond the preparation of future physician-scientists to encompass the larger issue of the scientific competency of the practicing physician. The first two Task Force recommendations address this challenge in asserting that *all* medical students should be sufficiently educated in the principles of clinical research to understand the peer-reviewed literature in their areas of specialization, to discuss research issues knowledgeably with a clinical investigator, and to explain relevant scientific or technical matters to a patient. In this, CRTF II embraced and heightened the visibility of recommendations of an AAMC expert panel led by Dennis Ausiello in 2000 that all physicians should achieve sufficient understanding of clinical research to be able to read the medical literature and evaluate the significance and implications of published discoveries and novel therapies in their own disciplines (Association of American Medical Colleges 2000b). Understandably, CRTF II reasoned that such exposure would also help encourage medical students to pursue clinical research careers.

Following AAMC's endorsement of the CRTF II report, the Liaison Committee for Medical Education (LCME) adopted a new accreditation standard for medical schools, while the ACGME introduced new language into its required core competencies consistent with the recommendation regarding graduate medical education. These two actions essentially adopt the task force's first two recommendations. When these new requirements are fully implemented, all medical students and residents should become more knowledgeable about clinical and translational research, thereby enhancing their capabilities as practitioners of medicine. Perhaps this greater exposure and deeper understanding will in time lead more students and residents to consider careers in clinical and translational research.

Consistent with AAMC's analyses, CRTF II agreed that there is an alarmingly high attrition rate of junior clinical research faculty investigators. For example, fewer than 40 percent of physicians receiving training awards through the NIH's (now superseded) Clinical Associate Physician Program had received any type of NIH grant funding within five years or more after the award (Association of American Medical Colleges 2006b, p. 22, information provided by Theodore Kotchen). Among the factors that appear to contribute to this attrition are insufficient training; complex and off-putting regulatory requirements; lack of scrupulously protected time for research; lack of program flexibility for women who wish to take time for bearing and rearing children; unavailability or inaccessibility of needed infrastructure; lack of consistently high-quality mentoring; the discouragingly lengthy time in training that seems to be required before one is successful in obtaining a first R01 grant (National Institutes of Health, Office of Extramural Research 2008); the seeming disadvantage of clinical research in NIH peer review; and the lure of greater financial rewards in full-time clinical practice. CRTF II proposed that these factors each be separately addressed by medical schools and teaching hospitals, including provision of benefits for maternity leave.

To stimulate the implementation and optimization of training pathways that will accelerate the progression of trainees to independence as physician-investigators (CRTF II, recommendation 5), the AAMC launched a new initiative by convening a group of medical school leaders who are interested in piloting novel educational and training pathways that encompass undergraduate and graduate medical education, as well as fellowship training, to produce clinical and translational physician-scientists capable of obtaining their first independent research funding while in their mid-thirties. This initiative has been dubbed "Accelerated Pathway to Independence for Clinician Scientists" (APICS).

The task force shared with many observers its concerns about recognizing the contributions of investigators as members of collaborative multidisciplinary teams, acknowledging that problem solving in biomedical science will increasingly rely on such teams. Promotion, advancement, and tenure decisions in medical schools have long required that candidates demonstrate "independence" in producing high-grade scholarship; in medical schools and research-intensive universities that demonstration has come to mean success in obtaining NIH R01 or comparable research funding. In such a system of evaluation, gaining appropriate recognition of faculty who provide essential, typically specialized support to research projects (e.g., statistical expertise, complex technological skills, and so on), and are neither "first" nor "last" authors but rather in the middle of the authorial pack in publication bylines, has long been a vexing challenge, and perhaps especially so in medical schools, where the "R01 culture" has become deeply embedded.

CRTF II emphasized the importance of documenting team member contributions, and such documentation is being facilitated by those journals that demand from each author of a manuscript, and then print, a description of his or her contribution to the study. Even more helpful would be widespread adoption by journals of the requirement that authors be listed alphabetically, as often happens in large team publications. Other important steps in the right direction, and also recommended by CRTF II, were the agreement of NIH (1) to begin listing in its CRISP (Computer Retrieval of Information on Scientific Projects) database of grant awards the names of co-investigators and the portions of the total award directed to their contributions to funded projects; and (2) to permit more than a single "principal investigator" on grant applications that can justify such designations.

The bottom line is that to recognize the role of multidisciplinary teams in biomedical and health sciences research, institutional tenure policies and practices, publication policies of the major journals, and NIH policies must all work together to support recognition and reward systems that no longer are fixated solely on the demonstration of "individual independence." After all, team science has long been a reality in the physical sciences, and universities, top-tier journals, and the Nobel Foundation, among others, have ably dealt with that reality.

Regarding infrastructure and administration, again echoing the prior task force, and consistent with the intent of the NIH's CTSA program, which had been announced during the task force's deliberations, CRTF II called for greater reliance on shared cores to support clinical research, including in bioinformatics, bioethics, protocol development, and community collaborations, and for sophisticated imaging, gene expression, proteomics technologies, and similar areas. Centralized leadership can best ensure appropriate investment in cutting-edge research infrastructure and in retention of key non-faculty research staff, who are often vital to the success of these programs. Where feasible, co-localization of infrastructure components should increase collaborative scientific interactions among clinical investigators (Heinig et al. 2007).

CRTF II also called for more effective linkages between academic medical centers, community physicians, practice-based networks, and community organizations to develop an "infrastructure" for clinical and public health research within communities. Establishing productive relationships is challenging for academics because they require institutions and investigative teams to treat communities as partners in, not subjects of, research. Attempts to develop community-based partnerships to support clinical research have been an important component of the CTSA program. For analysis of some of the formidable obstacles encountered, see Williams et al. 2008.)

CRTF II commended the progress made by the Department of Veterans Affairs in establishing a comprehensive, uniform electronic medical record system that supports both health care delivery and clinical and health services research. Despite a variety of other federal initiatives, and recurring political proclamations portraying the "electronic health record" (EHR) as a panacea for the problems that plague health care delivery, we have seen little if any follow-through on the critically important need to design EHRs that enable the entire gamut of clinical research, including health services and comparative effectiveness research. Despite the attention called to this issue as long ago as CRTF I, academic and nonacademic medical centers continue to implement EHR systems designed exclusively to meet the needs of hospital (or health care system) administration and finance.

CRTF II's strongest criticism was directed at the continued failure of the federal government to harmonize the thicket of regulations and procedures that address human research subjects protection (HRSP). The Department of Health and Human Services committed itself publicly to make HRSP regulations and policies of the NIH, the Food and Drug Administration, the Office of Human Research Protections, and other agencies more consistent; but despite evident commitment of the NIH (as part of its Roadmap), precious little has been accomplished across the agencies. For its part, the AAMC was a principal founder of the Association for the Accreditation of Human Research Protection Programs (AAHRPP, or "A-Harp"), which at this writing had accredited 159 organizations representing more than 750 individual entities involved in clinical research oversight.

Finally, from the examples the task force observed, many institutions had established major clinical research programs from substantial institutional commitments, while others without large resources had built competitive programs in narrower areas relevant to an area of expertise or central to the institution's mission. As has become evident from the enthusiasm and quality of applicants to the CTSA program (as of this writing, the NIH has funded thirty-eight CTSA consortia in twenty-three states), academic institutions are willing when appropriately challenged to garner extensive institutional support to finance comprehensive clinical research organizations. Notwithstanding, the academic medical community remains deeply concerned about the sustainability of these ambitious and often painstakingly negotiated programs under severely constrained NIH funding guidelines and flat-lined federal appropriations, and even more concerned for the fate of young scientists participating in the many clinical research and training initiatives begun in recent years (Heinig et al. 2007).

Conclusion: Protecting and Strengthening Clinical Research Integrity

In the AAMC's many efforts since 1997 to strengthen academic clinical research, consistent themes have been the recognition (1) that the revitalization of clinical research must begin with more robust education, training, and support, better nurturing, and ample protected time for clinical investigators; (2) that institutional structures and operations must be transformed to enable and facilitate the entire spectrum of clinical research and to accommodate better the demands of increasingly multidisciplinary scholarship; and, imperative for the success of the enterprise, (3) that academic medicine must reaffirm its commitment to the highest standards of professional integrity across its three core missions in order to sustain the public's trust. It is not surprising that both CRTFs invested the most effort in developing recommendations for investigator training and career development, including the need for change in institutional structure and infrastructure and in policies and practices relating to faculty recognition and reward. Noteworthy is the largely unplanned synchronicity and complementarity of AAMC task force recommendations with major NIH initiatives that were mutually reinforcing in their goals of strengthening and invigorating clinical research and training.

Since the mid-1960s—an era marked by enormous expansion of academic medicine's investment in and engagement with health care delivery and medical research; unprecedented advances in biomedical knowledge, technology, and understanding; a progressively aging population; and staggering increases in the nation's health care costs—it is disappointing and an indictment both of academic medicine and of society at large that the numbers of new physician-scientists (MD plus MD-PhD) competing for NIH research awards have remained essentially unchanged (see chapter 3). But perhaps this stagnation, or "failure to thrive," is not entirely surprising when we as a community have succeeded as much in encumbering clinical investigation as in facilitating it by neglecting a nurturing environment and weaving a thicket of increasingly complex regulations and procedural requirements around research involving human subjects or conceivably identifiable human materials (e.g., health information, tissue samples, genomic databases). We suggest that a society conducive to a robust clinical research enterprise requires from its members a greater sense of shared communal responsibility and respect for social goods and less focus on self.

Rigorous hypothesis-generating clinical and translational research and exploratory and confirmatory clinical trials, and the armamentarium of large-scale scientific efforts subsumed under health services research—the necessary components of a robust clinical research enterprise—are costly. And yet the Public Health Service agencies were largely flat-funded (or worse) between 2003–2008; during this interval the NIH lost nearly 14 percent of its 2003 purchasing power (Heinig et al. 2007). Although the infusion of research funding under the American Recovery and Reinvestment Act of 2009 is most gratifying, the United States and much of the world find themselves in dire financial and economic straits. Given the soaring U.S. budget deficit, it is difficult to predict federal budgets for biomedical and health sciences research, but we may at least hope for a sustained federal commitment to fiscal policies that avoid future boom-and-bust cycles.

A central challenge for the future is to preserve the social contract that has so generously supported U.S. academic scientific research and training while deferring much of the accountability for the conduct of that research and training to universities and academic medical centers. The biomedical sciences have benefited far more than other basic sciences from federal funding, given the appeal of the promise of better health and better management of disease and disability. Clinical research, as the Clinical Research Summit and others have noted, is central to fulfilling academic medicine's promise to the nation, and trust in the integrity of academic clinical research is the sine qua non of that social contract and fundamental to its continuation. The public expects our institutions to remain committed to honest stewardship of public funds, to protecting human research subjects, and to serving as sources of scientifically sound and disinterested information and advice on matters of public health. But at the same time, the public and its political representatives increasingly exhort academic institutions to partner with industry in promoting the transfer of new knowledge into useful application and in bringing social and economic benefits to their regions. Indeed, since NIH funding rarely if ever supports product development, interactions between medical scientist inventors and industry are the principal means by which new diagnostics, therapeutics, preventatives, and devices are developed and brought to market (Korn and Stanski 2006).

The resulting "conflict of public expectations" (Korn 2000) lies very much at the root of today's concerns with financial conflicts of interest in medical research, education, and clinical practice.

Public confidence in the integrity of academic clinical research has been shaken by repeated allegations of questionable practices and misbehavior by academic medical researchers, including the slanting or suppression of results from industry-sponsored clinical trials and failure by researchers and their institutions to disclose fully any financial self-interests that may be affected by their own research findings. The matter of identifying, managing, or eliminating financial conflicts of interest in federally funded biomedical research remains a daunting challenge. The AAMC alone and in partnership with the Association of American Universities has made major efforts to assist medical schools and teaching hospitals to deal with these issues and ensure that their relationships with industry are principled, scientifically sound, and transparent to the public (Association of American Medical Colleges and the Association of American Universities 2008). A thorough understanding of interactions with industry must be integrated into the training of every physician and physician-scientist, and the academic medicine community must make much greater efforts to educate the public about the processes by which scientific advancements are developed into products that prevent disease, mitigate suffering, and improve health.

To achieve the vision of the Clinical Research Summit and establish the robust clinical research enterprise that will play an essential role in addressing the many daunting problems that afflict our health care system will require many things. These include a national sense of purpose and commitment, sustained adequate funding for all components of the enterprise, rigorous scientific and ethical training of new investigators, and ongoing nurture and support of established investigators and the necessary infrastructure. But above all it will require from the entire medical profession a reaffirmation of and commitment to the highest ideals and standards of medical professionalism, and from medical scientists a recommitment to the principles, attitudes and behaviors of research integrity. Only by providing this affirmation will we be able to sustain the public's confidence and trust that in medical research as well as in practice, protecting the interest and well-being of our patients and human research participants is always our paramount responsibility.

14

Revitalizing the Nation's Physician-Scientist Workforce

THE ASSOCIATION OF PROFESSORS OF MEDICINE INITIATIVE

Andrew I. Schafer, MD

The academic medical community and the National Institutes of Health (NIH) have long been aware of jeopardy to the physician-scientist career path. As discussed elsewhere in this book, the number of physicians electing to pursue a primarily research-oriented career has declined in recent decades. The percentage of physicians engaged in research as their major professional activity in the United States decreased from a peak of 4.6 percent in 1985 to 1.8 percent in 2003. At the same time, the absolute number of physician-scientists dropped from a peak of about 23,000 in 1985 to 14,000 in 1995. This decline subsequently leveled off—a phenomenon that coincided with a doubling of the NIH budget between 1998 and 2003. Since 2003, however, the unpredictability of federal support for medical research, greatly exacerbated by the NIH budget's "undoubling," has led ever-increasing numbers of promising physicians to abandon their aspirations for research careers.

As described in the introduction, several important initiatives have been undertaken in recent years by organizations such as the NIH, the Institute of Medicine, and the Association of American Medical Colleges (see chapter 13) to attempt to reverse the decline in clinical investigators. Nevertheless, newer forces have now amplified concerns about the endangered physician-scientist workforce. These include important changes in the composition of the current generation of medical school graduates, particularly the dramatic influx of women, who appear to be not as interested as men in a physician-scientist career path, given the inflexibility of current academic promotion and tenure policies, as well as striking generational differences in priorities for work-life balance irrespective of gender.

To address these concerns, in 2006 the Association of Professors of Medicine (APM)—the organization of departments of internal medicine represented by chairs and appointed leaders at medical schools and affiliated teaching hospitals in the United States and Canada—initiated a concerted long-term effort to identify, develop, and help implement substantive but practical solutions that would ensure the survival and growth of the physician-scientist workforce of the next generation.

The APM Physician-Scientist Initiative was planned in linked phases. Phase I focused on the development of a strategy for evaluating the causes of the problem and the creation of a set of recommendations for revitalizing the physician-scientist workforce. This goal was achieved through a series of structured surveys and focus groups, which informed the agenda for a national consensus conference in 2007. Phase II was designed to expand and activate a coalition of key leadership organizations to move the agenda forward by developing a coordinated national strategy, as well as oversight of implementation of the action plan.

This chapter summarizes and comments on the results of national surveys and focus groups that were conducted in Phase I of the Physician-Scientist Initiative. It also presents the recommendations that emanated from a national consensus conference held in 2007. Finally, it provides an introduction to the action plan that was subsequently created.

Summary of Surveys and Focus Groups

In October 2006 an extensive survey was developed and distributed to leaders in academic medicine throughout North America to assess their opinions on the status of the physician-scientist workforce. Recipients included members of the APM, the Association of Specialty Professors, the Association of American Physicians, the American Society for Clinical Investigation, and the American Federation for Medical Research. Surveys were also distributed to all chairs of departments of internal medicine, psychiatry, pediatrics, obstetrics and gynecology, and dermatology. The survey was designed to elicit the respondents' opinions and views regarding attraction to and retention within the physician-scientist career path. The survey questioned respondents about current conditions and concerns as well as issues they encountered when they themselves entered the pipeline. In January 2007 a similar (but modified) survey was sent to all program directors of MD-PhD programs. Between October 2006 and May 2007 the APM held several facilitated, on-site, in-person focus groups with physician-scientist junior faculty and MD research fellows in training at six different institutions to explore contemporary views about career supports and barriers.

Detailed results of the survey data are available from the APM. The following represents a summary overview.

Demographics of Survey of Leaders in Academic Medicine

Of the total of 880 respondents, 85 percent were male. Their median years of obtaining their MD degree and their first faculty appointments were 1977 (range 1942–2002) and 1983 (range 1948–2004), respectively. Respondents conducted various types of research: basic laboratory research (32 percent); translational research (25 percent); clinical or patient-oriented research (32 percent); and health services research (8 percent).

The distribution of NIH funding ranks of the institutions at which the respondents were currently employed was as follows: first quartile (48 percent), second quartile (16 percent), third and fourth quartiles combined (16 percent).

Questions and Responses to Survey of Leaders in Academic Medicine

The following were some of the major questions asked, the distribution of responses to them, and the author's comments about interpretation.

1. What were the most important factors (positive or negative) that influenced your personal decision to pursue a physician-scientist career? (See figure 14.1.)
2. What do you think are the most important factors (positive or negative) that influence decisions by current and future trainees to pursue physician-scientist careers? (See figure 14.2.)

It is interesting to note that these established physician-scientist leaders of academic medicine recognized some generational shifts in the determinants of physicians' decisions to pursue research careers. "Innate curiosity," "positive physician-scientist role models," and "research experience during postgraduate training" ranked at the top of the list as motivating forces both for the established leaders themselves, as they recalled them, and in their perceptions about what drives the current generation of physicians to enter research careers. The second and third factors in particular seem to reflect the continued dominance of the "late bloomer" model of

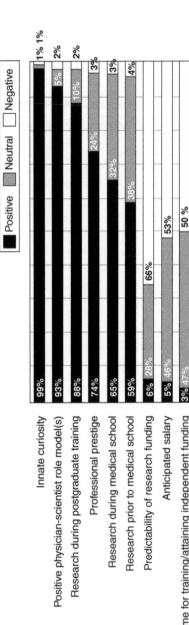

Figure 14.1. Responses to the question, "What were the most important factors (positive or negative) that influenced your personal decision to pursue a physician-scientist career?"

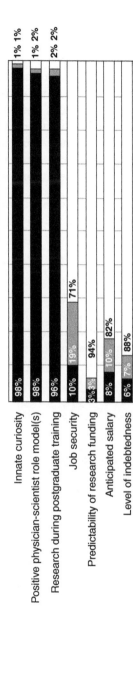

Figure 14.2. Responses to the question, "What do you think are the most important factors (positive or negative) that influence decisions by current and future trainees to pursue physician-scientist careers?"

physician-scientists (see chapter 10 by Kenneth Kaushansky), that is, those whose interest in research is sparked mainly after medical school.

After these three very positive influences, there is a divergence in the importance of factors that determine career decisions. For example, the "professional prestige" of being a physician-scientist was an important motivator for the established generation but not, in the opinion of these leaders, for recent medical school graduates (see figure 14.2). In contrast, job security, predictability of research funding, personal financial considerations (salary, level of indebtedness, time to completion of training), and a burdensome regulatory environment for research appear to have become much more powerful disincentives for the current generation.

3. What components of the local research environment do you think are most important for the success of young faculty?
   - *Utmost importance:*
   Mentoring (67%)
   Availability of adequate start-up support (57%)
   - *Very important:*
   Critical mass of investigators (58%)
   Access to strong trainees (55%)
   Research intensity of medical school (54%)
4. What were the most important factors (positive or negative) that influenced your decision to remain in a research career?
   - *Strongly positive:*
   Interest and enjoyment (84%)
   Innate curiosity (70%)
   Role models (53%)
   - *Weakly or strongly positive:*
   Opportunities to learn new science (91%)
   Professional prestige (82%)
   Leadership opportunities (79%)
   - *Weakly or strongly negative:*
   Unpredictable funding (94%)
   Indebtedness (83%)
   Salary (79%)

Opinions about this last question are particularly informative in light of a major consensus of the APM conference (discussed later in this chapter) that attrition of physician-scientists may be an even greater problem today than attracting young people into this career path.

5. What do you think is the relative likelihood of success of future initiatives to expand the physician-scientist workforce pipeline? (see figure 14.3)

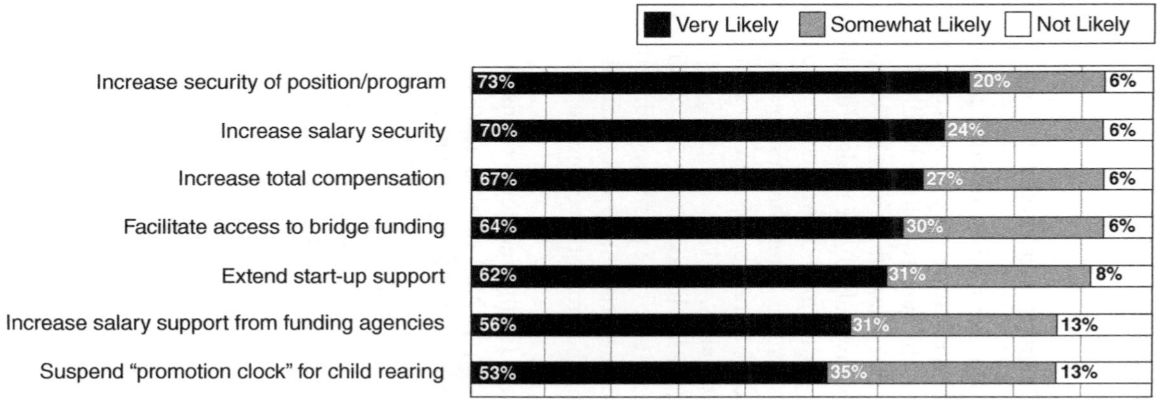

Figure 14.3. Responses to the question, "What do you think is the relative likelihood of future initiatives to expand the physician–scientist workforce pipeline?"

The striking finding here is that the respondents considered future initiatives related to personal finances the most likely to be successful in strengthening the physician-scientist career pipeline: increasing security of the position, increasing salary security, and increasing total compensation.

Subgroup Analysis of Responses to Survey

When we analyzed responses by subgroups of academic leaders, some interesting differences emerged. In terms of the local research environment, men perceived the research intensity of the medical school and access to strong trainees as more important than women. Women, however, placed more importance on the availability of bridge funding and flexibility in how professional effort is distributed. Women ranked a number of factors in retaining physician-scientists after the first few years more negatively than men. These included transition to other responsibilities within the current position, lifestyle, salary, and job security. They also had more positive opinions regarding the likelihood of success of some future initiatives, including increasing security for the position or program, promoting part-time pathways, extending start-up support, facilitating access to bridge funding, and suspending the promotion or tenure "clock" to accommodate child rearing.

Respondents who were faculty members of institutions that ranked in the first quartile nationally in NIH funding gave higher ratings than the other respondents to early research experience as a positive influence on their own careers. Respondents from institutions in the third and fourth quartiles for NIH funding more highly rated professional prestige and perceived requirements for a future academic leadership or administrative career as motivators to enter a physician-scientist career.

Survey of MD-PhD Program Directors

Forty-eight program directors responded to the survey, 56 percent of whom had MD degrees and 73 percent PhD degrees. The median duration of program directorship was four years (ranging from one to twenty-five years), and the median year of first faculty appointment was 1986 (range 1965–1998).

The major conclusions of this survey, which was modified from that sent to academic physician-scientist leaders, were the following. First, there was strong consensus that graduates of combined MD-PhD degree programs should become physician-scientists. Second, respondents suggested that to be a successful physician-scientist requires greater than 50 percent professional effort devoted to research. Third, respondents cited several future initiatives as being most likely to succeed in strengthening the physician-scientist career path: increasing salary security (64%); increasing position security (58%); creating part-time pathways (58%); extending start-up support (58%); and reprioritizing medical school admission criteria to favor applicants interested in research careers (56%).

Extending the length of MD-PhD training emerged in multiple questions as a significant disincentive to entering the physician-scientist career pathway.

Some of the opinions of MD-PhD program directors expressed in this survey contrast strikingly with those of MD-PhD students themselves in a survey that was conducted independently and contemporaneously, and published in *Academic Medicine* (Ahn et al. 2007). While their program directors felt that greater than 50 percent professional effort directed at research is needed to become a successful physician-scientist, 41 percent of the MD-PhD students did not agree with the definition of a physician-scientist as someone who performs research as his or her primary professional activity. While the program directors reached strong consensus that MD-PhD graduates should become physician-scientists, almost half of the students indicated that they did not wish to become physician-scientists as currently defined. This was because they did not intend to conduct research as their primary professional activity. Significant differences like these in the views of faculty program directors and their students have important potential implications. They illuminate generational disagreements about the degree of commitment to research that is needed to become a productive physician-scientist. Indeed they also suggest that MD-PhD programs may not be as successful as widely assumed in their mission to train physician-scientists.

Summary of Focus Groups

Seven facilitated focus groups with junior physician-scientists (training fellows, instructors, assistant professors, and a few associate professors) were conducted onsite at six institutions: the University of Pennsylvania School of Medicine, Johns Hopkins University School of Medicine, Mount Sinai School of Medicine, University of Minnesota School of Medicine, Jefferson Medical College of Thomas Jefferson University, and Harvard Medical School–Beth Israel Deaconess Medical Center. While opinions often reflected the unique characteristics of each institution and, to some extent, distinctive local issues, some overarching conclusions could be drawn from these discussions.

The majority of participants chose a research career because they considered science to be exciting, intellectually stimulating, and fun. Furthermore, for some participants, physician-scientist careers were thought to provide a good balance and alternative to patient care as well as day-to-day independence and flexibility. Consistently the greatest worry of these young physician-scientists is the constant drumbeat of pressure over research funding. There was a clear realization that one is "in the game" only as long as the funding continues. Largely because of the inevitable burnout from chasing research support, roughly one-third of participants had already begun to think of changing or altering their career paths. Most participants viewed difficulties in keeping people in the pipeline and helping them make the transition from career development awards to independent funding as the most daunting problem facing the future physician-scientist workforce.

Recommendations for Revitalizing the Physician-Scientist Workforce

The APM Physician-Scientist Initiative Consensus Conference, "Revitalization of the Nation's Physician-Scientist Workforce," was held in Washington, D.C., in November 2007. The conference assembled an invited group of about one hundred leaders of the academic, medical, and research communities. These included representatives from the various governing bodies that influence and fund biomedical research; thought leaders and experts on various facets of the physician-scientist workforce problem; and a number of young physician-scientists to provide firsthand present-day perspectives on issues facing them. A list of participants is included at the end of this chapter.

The conference was interactive in format, with targeted breakout groups focused on specific aspects of the physician-scientist career path. The full group debated and discussed additional opportunities to strengthen the physician-scientist career pipeline through both increased entry and improved retention. A total of thirty highly specific recommendations emanated from the conference breakout sessions and general group discussions. Following the conference, the participants provided a more detailed analytical assessment, prioritizing, commenting on, and finally editing the recommendations to create a more sharply focused action plan.

The conference produced four major, overarching recommendations to revitalize the physician-scientist workforce, with a number of specific recommendations under each of them. Each recommendation is targeted at specific constituencies (e.g., the NIH, foundations, medical schools, academic medical centers). They can be summarized as follows:

1. *Attention and Resources Should Be Directed at Repairing the "Leaking" Physician-Scientist Pipeline.* Traditionally physician-scientists have been developed en masse, with institutions launching numerous careers in the hope of retaining a relatively low yield of successful independent investigators.
   - Institutions should consolidate their focus on accommodating, retaining, and then fully supporting the most promising physician-scientist faculty members with sufficient and more stable resources, competitive salaries, mentoring, and protected time for research.
   - NIH should optimize its mechanisms of support for the career development (K) award, including increased salary support, flexibility in award duration to accommodate time out for family responsibilities, and financial support for mentors commensurate with effort. With thoughtful guidance and peer review, NIH should implement a mechanism to terminate clearly nonproductive K awards, but without discouraging high-risk innovative research by committed trainees.
   - NIH should substantially increase support for first-time R awards, since a major vulnerable point in the pipeline occurs in the transition to independence.
   - NIH should direct funds to study and monitor its investigator workforce, particularly tracking applicants over time, analyzing the effectiveness of its grant mechanisms, and studying the impact of policy changes on career decisions. Academic societies should track data on trends among physician-scientists who join the biotechnology and pharmaceutical industries.
2. *Major Changes Should Be Made to the Contemporary Approach to Mentoring Physician-Scientists.* The success of physician-scientists today requires institutionally mandated, career-long, multidimensional guidance and support by teams of skilled mentors who contribute dedicated effort to this activity.
   - Institutions should create and implement formalized mentoring programs for physician-scientists that incorporate several contemporary facets.

- Mentees may require team-based mentoring by groups of mentors who have complementary skills and insights into various aspects of a physician-scientist career.
  - Institutions should organize multigenerational mentoring groups to acknowledge and reconcile the striking generational differences in attitudes toward work-life balance and controllable lifestyles.
  - Institutions should ensure that mentors reflect the diversity of the workforce and that they are trained in approaches to mentoring junior faculty of different genders, races, and ethnicities.
- Mentoring programs should include formalized training in career negotiation and tracks, grant writing and management, and presentations and publications as well as scientific guidance.
- Institutions should provide formalized training in mentoring skills and establish evaluation systems to ensure effective mentoring.
- Mentors should receive financial support commensurate with professional effort from the institution and/or granting agency.
- NIH should expand mentoring awards in scope and amount for senior physician-scientists through the K series to support and enhance dedicated mentoring of junior physician-scientists, enabling better utilization of the time and effort of many senior researchers, and potentially freeing up additional RO1-type awards for junior and mid-career investigators.

3. *Institutions Should Actively Promote the Advancement and Minimize the Attrition of Women in Physician-Scientist Careers.* The demographics of medical school graduates are rapidly transforming, with female graduates expected to constitute the majority in the coming years. Academic medicine must take advantage of this opportunity to expand the physician-scientist workforce to include female faculty. Yet women physicians generally find research careers less appealing and accommodating than men.
   - Institutions should ensure that men and women of equal academic standing receive equivalent protected time, start-up packages, bridge funding, space, and access to other resources.
   - Institutions should substantially increase the flexibility of time-based review in the promotion process and in the tenure clock for investigators who need additional time to move to successful independent funding.
   - Institutions should aggressively support the provision of easily accessible on-site child care, the development of lab schools, and other initiatives that equalize opportunities for women to succeed as physician-scientists, remain productive in physician-scientist careers, and attain leadership positions in academic medicine.

4. *The Physician-Scientist Workforce Should Be Strengthened by Earlier and Better-Coordinated Efforts to Identify and Prepare Successful Future Investigators with a More Enduring Commitment to Research Careers.*

   • Universities should broaden the focus of undergraduate premedical education curricula to place greater emphasis on the physical sciences and quantitative skills, molecular biology and genetics, biostatistics, and ethics. In turn, the Association of American Medical Colleges should alter the Medical College Admission Test to reflect the curriculum changes.

   • Medical schools should partner with the premedical adviser community to promote the physician-scientist pathway to undergraduate students.

   • Resource-intensive medical schools should alter their admissions committee culture to accommodate more applicants with strong research interests, including special subcommittees that make decisions related to students interested in research.

   • Research-intensive medical schools should focus interest and resources on medical student research by providing a full-year of research and stipends for approved full-time student researchers.

Implementation of Recommendations

Implementation of these recommendations will be challenging. In many cases it will involve paradigm shifts in how medical schools and academic medical centers currently function under time-honored conventions and protocols for faculty development. It will also involve well-coordinated and integrated initiatives by government funding agencies, foundations, philanthropies, regulatory bodies, and educational institutions that have not traditionally functioned in cooperative ways. To begin the process, the APM and the Association of American Medical Colleges (AAMC) have worked together to advance many of the proposed changes.

AAMC-APM Workshop

To follow up on the AAMC Clinical Research Task Forces I and II (see chapter 13 by David Korn and Stephen Heinig) and the APM Physician-Scientist Initiative, the AAMC and APM jointly convened a workshop on the physician-scientist workforce at the AAMC Annual Meeting in October 2008. A predominant outcome of the conference was strong consensus about the importance of developing innovative programs to provide early and sustained immersion of prospective young physician-scientists in medical research, even calling for a "Head Start"–type initiative during the high school years (or earlier). At the same time, it was felt that current medical school and postgraduate clinical training curricula create a protracted interlude without meaningful research exposure, which often extinguishes a potential young physician-scientist's early interest in a research career. Therefore there was a renewed call for the accrediting organizations (the Liaison Committee on Medical Education and the Accreditation Council for Graduate Medical Education) to incorporate substantive research exposure in their accreditation standards. Finally, since virtually every academically oriented medical organization today recognizes the vital importance of physician-scientists, the AAMC-APM conference called for a cohesive and coordinated platform for gathering data, sharing information and best practices between different specialties, and joint strategic planning to ensure the survival of a vibrant physician-scientist workforce.

Appendix

Acknowledgments

The following sponsors provided support for the APM conference and physician-scientist initiative: National Institutes of Health (National Heart, Lung and Blood Institute as lead institute; Office of the Director, National Cancer Institute; National Center for Complementary and Alternative Medicine; National Center on Minority Health and Health Disparities; National Eye Institute; National Institute of Allergy and Infectious Diseases; National Institute of Arthritis and Musculoskeletal and Skin Diseases; National Institute of Biomedical Imaging and Bioengineering; National Institute of Child Health and Human Development; National Institute of Diabetes and Digestive and Kidney Diseases; National Institute of Environmental Health Sciences; National Institute of Mental Health); Burroughs Wellcome Fund; Doris Duke Charitable Foundation; Robert Wood Johnson Foundation; American Academy of Allergy, Asthma and Immunology; American Gastroenterological Association; American Society of Clinical Oncology; and American Society of Nephrology.

Judy A. Shea, PhD, professor of medicine at the University of Pennsylvania, was instrumental in designing, conducting, and analyzing the surveys and focus groups.

Participants in the APM Physician-Scientist Consensus Conference

Titles and institutional affiliations are as of the time of the conference. Planning Committee members are marked with an asterisk.

Andrew I. Schafer, MD, Conference Chair*; President, American Society of Hematology; Chair, Department of Medicine, Weill Cornell Medical College

Jaimo Ahn, MD, PhD, Resident, Department of Orthopedic Surgery, University of Pennsylvania School of Medicine

Duane Alexander, MD, Director, National Institute of Child Health and Human Development, National Institutes of Health

Barbara M. Alving, MD, Director, National Center for Research Resources, National Institutes of Health

Olaf S. Andersen, MD, Past President, National MD-PhD Directors Association; Professor of Physiology and Biophysics, Weill Cornell Medical College

James M. Anderson, MD, PhD, Chair, Department of Cell and Molecular Physiology, University of North Carolina School of Medicine

Nancy C. Andrews, MD, PhD*, President-Elect, American Society for Clinical Investigation; Dean, Duke University School of Medicine

Mark W. Babyatsky, MD*, Vice Chair of Education, Department of Medicine, Mount Sinai School of Medicine

Timothy R. Billiar, MD, Chair, Department of Surgery, University of Pittsburgh School of Medicine

Lawrence F. Brass, MD, PhD, President, National MD-PhD Directors Association, University of Pennsylvania School of Medicine

William J. Bremner, MD, PhD, President, Association of Professors of Medicine; Chair, Department of Medicine, University of Washington School of Medicine

Ann J. Brown, MD, Associate Vice Dean for Faculty Development, Duke University School of Medicine

Robert M. Califf, MD, Vice Chancellor for Clinical Research, Director, Translational Medicine Institute, Duke University School of Medicine

Andrew M. Cameron, MD, PhD, Assistant Professor, Department of Surgery, Johns Hopkins University School of Medicine

Henry Chang, MD, Medical Officer, Division of Blood Diseases and Resources, National Heart, Lung and Blood Institute, National Institutes of Health

Virginia W. Chang, MD, PhD, Assistant Professor, Departments of Medicine and Sociology, University of Pennsylvania

Barry S. Coller, MD, David Rockefeller Professor of Medicine, Physician in Chief, Rockefeller University

William F. Crowley, Jr., MD*, Chair, Board of Directors, Clinical Research Forum, Harvard Medical School and Massachusetts General Hospital

Pamela Davis, MD, PhD, Dean, Case Western Reserve University School of Medicine

Prabhjot S. Dhadialla, MD-PhD Student, Weill Cornell Medical College and Rockefeller University

Clemente Diaz, MD, Chair, Department of Pediatrics, University of Puerto Rico

Howard B. Dickler, MD*, Director for Clinical Research, Association of American Medical Colleges

Mark Donowitz, MD, President, American Gastroenterological Association; LeBoff Professor of Medicine, Johns Hopkins University School of Medicine

Stephen G. Emerson, MD, PhD, President, Haverford College

David M. Engman, MD, PhD, President-Elect, National MD-PhD Program Directors Association; Professor of Pathology, Northwestern University Feinberg School of Medicine

Stephen D. Fihn, MD, Head, Division of General Internal Medicine, University of Washington School of Medicine

John N. Forrest Jr., MD, Professor of Medicine, Director, Office of Student Research, Yale University School of Medicine

John J. Frangioni, MD, PhD, Associate Professor of Medicine and Radiology, Harvard Medical School and Beth Israel Deaconess Medical Center

Michael J. Friedlander, PhD, Chair, Department of Neuroscience, Baylor College of Medicine

Naomi K. Fukagawa, MD, PhD, Professor of Medicine, University of Vermont College of Medicine

Leo T. Furcht, MD, Immediate Past President, Federation of American Societies for Experimental Biology; Head, Department of Laboratory Medicine and Pathology, University of Minnesota School of Medicine

William R. Galey Jr., PhD*, Director of Graduate and Medical Programs, Howard Hughes Medical Institute

John I. Gallin, MD, Director, Clinical Center, National Institutes of Health

Gary H. Gibbons, MD, Director, Cardiovascular Research Institute, Morehouse School of Medicine

Henry N. Ginsberg, MD, Director, Irving Institute for Clinical and Translational Research, Columbia University College of Physicians and Surgeons

Pascal J. Goldschmidt, MD, Dean, University of Miami Leonard M. Miller School of Medicine

Michelle Ng Gong, MD, Assistant Professor of Medicine, Mount Sinai School of Medicine

Michael R. Grever, MD, Chair, Department of Medicine, Ohio State University College of Medicine

Mary Beth E. Hamel, MD, Deputy Editor, *New England Journal of Medicine;* Associate Professor of Medicine, Harvard Medical School and Beth Israel Deaconess Medical Center

Robert I. Handin, MD, Executive Vice Chair, Department of Medicine, Harvard Medical School and Brigham and Women's Hospital

Donna E. Hansel, MD, PhD, Assistant Professor of Anatomic Pathology, Cleveland Clinic Lerner College of Medicine of Case Western University

Margaret K. Hostetter, MD, Chair, Department of Pediatrics, Yale University School of Medicine

J. Larry Jameson, MD, PhD, Dean, Northwestern University Feinberg School of Medicine

Wishwa N. Kapoor, MD, Director, Institute of Clinical Research Education, University of Pittsburgh School of Medicine

Kenneth Kaushansky, MD, President-Elect, American Society of Hematology; Chair, Department of Medicine, University of California at San Diego School of Medicine

Talmadge E. King Jr., MD, Chair, Department of Medicine, University of California at San Francisco School of Medicine

Gary A. Koretzky, MD, PhD, Chief, Division of Rheumatology, University of Pennsylvania School of Medicine

Alan M. Krensky, MD, Director, Office of Portfolio Analysis and Strategic Initiatives, National Institutes of Health

Joel E. Kupersmith, MD, Chief Research and Development Officer, Veterans Health Administration, Department of Veterans Affairs

Beth Levine, MD, Chief, Division of Infectious Diseases, University of Texas Southwestern Medical Center at Dallas

Wendy S. Levinson, MD, Chair, Department of Medicine, University of Toronto School of Medicine

Timothy J. Ley, MD, Professor of Medicine, Washington University School of Medicine

Allen S. Lichter, MD, Executive Vice President and Chief Executive Officer, American Society of Clinical Oncology

Stuart L. Linas, MD*, Professor of Medicine, University of Colorado School of Medicine

Nancy Maizels, PhD, Professor of Immunology and Biochemistry, Director, Molecular Medicine Program, University of Washington School of Medicine

Justin McArthur, MBBS, Vice Chair, Department of Neurology, Johns Hopkins University School of Medicine

Ravindra L. Mehta, MD, Associate Chair for Clinical Affairs, Department of Medicine, University of California at San Diego School of Medicine

Juanita L. Merchant, MD, PhD*, Professor of Internal Medicine, University of Michigan Medical School

Elizabeth Myers, PhD*, Program Officer, Medical Research Program, Doris Duke Charitable Foundation

Elizabeth G. Nabel, MD, Director, National Heart, Lung and Blood Institute, National Institutes of Health

Eric G. Neilson, MD, Chair, Department of Medicine, Vanderbilt University School of Medicine

Enid Neptune, MD, Assistant Professor of Medicine, Johns Hopkins University School of Medicine

Freddy Nguyen*, President, American Physician Scientists Association, MD-PhD Student, University of Illinois at Urbana-Champaign

James C. Oates, MD*, President, American Federation for Medical Research; Associate Professor of Medicine, Medical University of South Carolina

J. Carl Oberholtzer, MD, PhD, Office of Centers, Training, and Resources, National Cancer Institute, National Institutes of Health

Aimee S. Payne, MD, PhD, Assistant Professor of Dermatology, University of Pennsylvania School of Medicine

Roger M. Perlmutter, MD, Executive Vice President for Research and Development, Amgen

Philip A. Pizzo, MD, Dean, Stanford University School of Medicine

Kenneth S. Polonsky, MD, Chair, Department of Internal Medicine, Washington University School of Medicine

Jonathan I. Ravdin, MD, Chair, Department of Medicine, University of Minnesota School of Medicine

Albert Reece, MD, PhD, Dean, University of Maryland School of Medicine

Robert R. Rich, MD, Senior Vice President and Dean, University of Alabama at Birmingham School of Medicine

Griffin P. Rodgers, MD, Director, National Institute of Diabetes, Digestive and Kidney Diseases, National Institutes of Health

Matthew Randall Rosengart, MD, MPH, Assistant Professor of Surgery, University of Pittsburgh School of Medicine

Paul B. Rothman, MD*, Chair, Department of Internal Medicine, University of Iowa Carver College of Medicine

Christopher Rowley, MD, MPH, Instructor, Department of Medicine, Harvard Medical School and Beth Israel Deaconess Medical Center

Norka Ruiz Bravo, PhD, Director, Office of Extramural Research, National Institutes of Health

Barbara L. Schuster, MD, Past President, Association of Professors of Medicine; Professor of Internal Medicine, Wright State University School of Medicine

Victor L. Schuster, MD, Chair, Department of Medicine, Albert Einstein College of Medicine

Alan L. Schwartz, MD, PhD, Chair, Department of Pediatrics, Washington University School of Medicine

Robert S. Sherwin, MD, Director, Yale Center for Clinical Investigation, Yale University School of Medicine

David E. Steward, MD, President-Elect, Association of Professors of Medicine; Chair, Department of Medicine, Southern Illinois University School of Medicine

Nancy S. Sung, PhD*, Founding Chair, Health Research Alliance; Senior Program Officer, Burroughs Wellcome Fund

Nancy J. Tarbell, MD, Chief, Pediatric Radiation Oncology Unit, Harvard Medical School and Massachusetts General Hospital

Myron L. Weisfeldt, MD*, Chair, Department of Medicine, Johns Hopkins University School of Medicine

Stephanie Weiss, PhD, Medical Student, Cleveland Clinic Lerner College of Medicine of Case Western Reserve University

Donald E. Wesson, MD*, Vice Dean, Texas A&M University College of Medicine

Edward J. Wing, MD, Chair, Department of Medicine, Warren Alpert Medical School of Brown University

Janet Woodcock, MD, Deputy Commissioner and Chief Medical Officer, U.S. Food and Drug Administration

Mark L. Zeidel, MD*, Chair, Department of Medicine, Harvard Medical School and Beth Israel Deaconess Medical Center

15

A Half Century of Clinical Research

David G. Nathan, MD

It seems fitting to end this book with the personal reflections of one of the most influential physician-scientists of our time. They capture his lifelong romance with clinical research; the endless cascade of answers to clinical questions begetting new questions; the continuous cycling of research in both directions between bedside and bench, inspired by an insatiable curiosity. Most important, the essay reflects the unfettered and unabashed joy and pride of a great mentor who revels in the achievements of his students.

David G. Nathan has been a legendary chief of hematology, chair of the Department of Pediatrics, and physician in chief of Children's Hospital, Boston, and the Harvard Medical School. He then served with distinction as president of the Dana Farber Cancer Institute. Among his most notable original contributions in his work with trainees who would later constitute a virtual "who's who" of American hematology include elucidation of the molecular basis of thalassemia, the development of DNA-based prenatal diagnostic testing, pioneering iron chelation therapy, and major additions to our current understanding of hematopoiesis. Of particular relevance to this volume, David Nathan was asked by Harold Varmus, then head of the NIH, to chair the NIH Director's Panel on Clinical Research, which between 1995 and 1997 developed groundbreaking recommendations to promote clinical research and clinical investigators (Nathan and Wilson 2003).

In his introduction of David Nathan as the 2006 recipient of the Kober Medal of the Association of American Physicians, Edward Benz, himself a renowned physician-scientist and a student of Nathan's, noted that Nathan

had and continues "to launch and nurture the careers of an incredibly large
number of extraordinary scholars and leaders whose own contributions di-
rectly amplify David's" and who, "in turn, have produced and are even now
producing leaders." Benz concluded that "at a time when we fear the demise
of the physician-scientist and physician-scholar," David Nathan "is person-
ally keeping the pipeline flowing" (Benz 2007).—Andrew I. Schafer, MD

When my father, who dearly wanted to be a physician and had actually
been admitted to the Harvard Medical School in 1920, told my grandfather that he planned to go to medical school, the splendid Victorian gentle-
man whom I intensely admired categorically intoned, "No son of mine is
going to be a fake and a phony who comes to your house, drinks your cof-
fee and can't do a damned thing for you." Which explains why my father
dutifully entered a branch of the family business. My grandfather's views
were forged in an era when, as Paul Starr describes in his superb account
The Social Transformation of American Medicine (Starr 1982), surgeons provided very much to patients, while physicians, including internists, pediatricians, and general practitioners, had little to offer other than sympathy.

My father's love of medicine never diminished, and I felt its pressure
throughout my middle and high school years. Yet when I arrived at Harvard College in 1947, I determined to become an English teacher. That
decision upset my father no end. He had graduated from Harvard with
a BS in chemistry, a far more practical subject, he thought, than English
literature. Nonetheless, I persisted and wrote a tedious thesis on Matthew
Arnold, a Victorian poet. I realized, however, in my sophomore year, that
while I affected the image of an English teacher, especially the accoutre-
ments, including a tweed jacket with leather elbow patches and a pipe,
I singularly lacked the talent. My parsing skills were no better than my
football performance; hence I applied to Harvard Medical School when
I realized that my deepest interest lay in what I might be able to do for
people in need. That awakening probably represented the influence of my
mother, a Simmons College graduate in social work, who had directed the
Red Cross Home Service in World War II. When I was admitted, my father
was overjoyed, and my mother beamed as well.

When I entered Harvard Medical School, I wanted to become an internist and start a clinic for poor residents of East Cambridge, where I lived. I
envisaged a group practice of salaried physicians. The concept was novel
at the time, and it probably influenced the school to admit me even though
my academic performance at Harvard College, though reasonable, was
scarcely noteworthy. That goal persisted until midway through the second

year, when I saw a patient with hepatic coma and a flapping tremor on the wards of the Boston City Hospital, where William B. Castle was physician in chief. When I asked the chief resident what had happened, he told me that the patient, who had alcoholic cirrhosis, had just eaten a large meal and had gone into coma shortly thereafter. He didn't know the reason, but some evidence gathered in Europe suggested that the coma might be due to an elevation of blood ammonia, the latter derived from the proteins in the meal. At that time blood ammonia was very difficult to measure, and the resident was not sure of the etiology. Perhaps because of my interest in English mystery stories, this example of endogenous poisoning was fascinating and led me to pursue the problem first in the Department of Pathology and then in Biochemistry.

The curriculum at the time was open on Tuesday, Thursday, and Saturday afternoons. Lee Rodkey, an assistant professor of biochemistry, gave me a bench in his lab, and we set about to develop a method for measuring blood ammonia. In my fourth year Lee and I published that paper, and several hospitals adopted the method in their clinical laboratories. As I finger its yellowing pages now, I accept that it is not very important, but that paper and the work that led to it absolutely turned me on to a career in clinical research. It taught me that I wanted to find out why patients are sick and to try to find new ways to help them. Many years later I concluded that the research bug should bite at the medical student level or before. After an involvement in the training of physician-scientists that has lasted almost fifty years, it is clear to me that the most successful are those who began "the life" in college or medical school. MD-PhD programs are probably most valuable because of their timing (to say nothing of their financial benefits).

Between 1955 and 1956 I was an intern in medicine at the then Peter Bent Brigham Hospital, a Dickensian institution with large open wards connected to a long corridor. The wards and the corridor were freezing in the winter and stifling in the summer. There was little or no privacy. The air was filled with groans, coughs, and flatus. I will never forget two patients in adjoining beds, one a luetic, the other an alcoholic, both thoroughly demented. One night the luetic decided to teach the alcoholic mathematics. Suddenly a cry rang out in the night. The luetic was screaming: "I'll never teach him calculus again. He just urinated in my shoes!"

That evening was not atypical. Interns worked every other night and weekend for $25 a month. At night we ran a thirty-bed ward alone with a student nurse and vaguely supervised by a senior resident. An experienced head nurse might get $4,000 a year. The patients, who paid a bed rate of about $30 a day, remained in the hospital for weeks and thereby gave me an education in the natural course of disease and effects of treatment that is presently unobtainable.

Though the infrastructure of the Brigham was deficient, the level of clinical research was extraordinary. Cardiac catheterization and cardiac valve surgery were pioneered in that fetid environment. The treatment of kidney failure by dialysis and transplantation both began there while I was a house officer. Moreover, the clinical training was in the hands of superb physicians in private practice like Samuel A. Levine, the great cardiologist of his era. The balance of science and art in medicine was inspiring to a young man groping for a career, and the contact with these mentors proved invaluable.

A career in clinical research mixed with patient care and teaching heavily attracted me, but I would never have had a viable opportunity had the United States not been involved in military campaigns. The doctor draft, reinitiated by the Korean conflict, mandated military service after internship. Suddenly I had to make a choice. I could join the medical corps of one of the armed services or the United States Public Health Service as a commissioned officer in the newly opened and glittering Clinical Center (now the Magnesen Clinical Center) of the National Institutes of Health. With a wife and two children in tow, I quickly chose the latter. My assignment, and that of two of my most distinguished classmates, Tom Waldmann and Sherman Weissman, was to the Metabolism Service of the National Cancer Institute in the laboratory of the late Nathaniel I. Berlin, an experimental hematologist. That's when I learned about the power of military rank. When I informed Berlin that I wanted to study ammonia metabolism in liver disease, he folded his gnome-like frame into a government-issued desk chair, rocked back and forth like a Jewish Buddha, and, pointing to the figurative two stripes on my sleeve and to the four on his, explained, "That difference is why you are going to be a hematologist and not an expert in liver disease." I believe I may be one of very few academic hematologists who was ordered into the field.

I actually solved the dilemma of field choice by compromise. By day I worked for Berlin on measurements of red blood cell production and lifespan in various kinds of leukemia while I participated in the development of the first combination chemotherapy for those diseases. In the evening I shared a lab with the late Kenneth Warren, another former medical school classmate, who was also interested in ammonia. The result was a collection of papers in *Blood* and the *Journal of Clinical Investigation* that brought me an invitation to return to the Brigham in 1958, first as a senior resident in medicine and then as a junior staff member in the hematology division under the watchful eye of Frank H. Gardner.

For seven years I was able to take advantage of the flow of fascinating patients in that urban academic community hospital. The facilities remained cramped and obsolete, but the patients provided nonpareil opportunities for care, teaching, and research. In fact most of the patients who were the subjects of my research were those for whose care I was responsible. They trusted me, and I knew that I would never willingly abuse that trust. Nonetheless, my research plans, though discussed carefully by the hematology division members in our weekly meeting, were not presented to third parties such as an institutional review board (IRB). Thus neither my ideas nor anyone else's were ever subjected to dispassionate peer review. Although I was far less burdened by administrative delay mediated by "chronophages," in the words of the late Judah Folkman, my ethical decisions were simply too inbred. We needed the dispassionate IRB system, the brilliantly conceived process instituted in the 1970s but now hobbled by mission creep (Gunsalus, Bruner, and Burbules 2006).

Diseases of the red blood cells became the focus of my research. By studying red cell production in renal failure and in anephric patients, we were able to prove that there must be extra-renal sources of erythropoietin. A patient with thalassemia intermedia had entered my life during my senior residency. He was thought to have metastatic cancer, but I suspected that the huge round infiltrates in his lungs were explants of bone marrow. I was right and became hooked on that fascinating disease. The late Robert Gunn, then a medical student, and I showed that the clinical consequences of thalassemia are due to unbalanced rather than deficient globin chain synthesis. Then Tom Gabuzda and I demonstrated the important role of fetal hemoglobin in the survival of thalassemic red cells.

All of this attracted the attention of the late William Castle, the tall, laconic, and humorous chief of Harvard's Thorndike medical service at the Boston City Hospital. Castle was an icon in American academic medicine and for good reason. A superb physician himself, Castle had a gargantuan knowledge of the medical literature, employed uncomplicated laboratory techniques to answer complex scientific questions, wrote fluidly, and was devoted to the training of physician-scientists. There was simply no mentor like him. He encouraged two of his best young faculty members, the late Rudi Schmid and Jim Jandl, to help me solve tough scientific problems.

Careers are often made by chance events that are beyond one's control. Frank Gardner and the late Louis K. Diamond, the great pediatric hematologist at the Children's Hospital, had struck up a collaboration. Diamond became interested in my investigation of the basis of acquired and congenital red blood cell diseases and, through one of his most brilliant trainees, the late Frank A. Oski, began to send me curious cases. Though I knew little or no pediatrics, I had Oski—who was both a fine investigator and a superb pediatrician—as a collaborator. Together we attacked a host of congenital red cell problems from pyruvate kinase deficiency to leaky red cell membranes. After Oski left for the University of Pennsylvania, we continued our collaboration. The work excited me, and I began to wonder why I was in internal medicine rather than pediatrics.

Frank Gardner saw that I was getting restless and, hoping to keep me on the reservation, promised to expand my space. To do so he bought a trailer and hired a construction crane to lower it next to our laboratories. In it there was room for my office and a liquid scintillation counter. I was grateful, but my mind was constantly veering toward those pediatric patients with their fascinating red cell disorders. Suddenly my situation became much clearer. Gardner decided to leave the Brigham and go to the University of Pennsylvania. At the same time, Diamond, close to retirement, announced that he was leaving Children's to be nearer his family in California. Within days of his decision, the late Charles A. Janeway, then chief of medicine at the Children's Hospital, called to invite me to discuss my future with him.

The first meeting with Janeway settled the matter. He offered me an opportunity to come to Children's to establish a hematology division that would focus on the patients and use modern scientific methods to explore diagnoses and new treatments. He would provide some equipment, such as a fraction collector that was gathering dust in another laboratory. The rest of the support would have to come from grants and gifts, for which I would have to apply.

I liked the deal. I was being given responsibility, and I was used to providing for my own efforts. I didn't expect a start-up package. The idea was unknown to me. Furthermore, I simply wanted to work for Janeway. I admired him on sight. He was extraordinarily intelligent, humane, devoted to clinical research, and endowed with the understanding that we all have our weaknesses and strengths. An effective division chief, he taught me, must determine the strengths of faculty members and try to avoid their weaknesses. Dr. Castle put it another way. "Don't," he warned, "get into the ring with Joe Louis. He will beat you up. You are a clinical investigator, not a basic scientist. Stick with your patients. You can win with them. Let the basic scientists work with model organisms." Castle was, above all, an adherent of the view of Alexander Pope: "The proper study of mankind is man."

The challenge of Janeway's offer was very real. Years before, following the untimely death of Soma Weiss, his chief at the Brigham, he had transferred his laboratory and clinical interests to Children's Hospital and had become a pediatrician. He assured me that I could do the same. But I was filled with doubt. Janeway was a remarkably bright man. It was not clear to me that I could learn enough pediatrics to be acceptable to my colleagues in an institution as advanced as Children's. And none of my friends in internal medicine were encouraging. They all warned me that I would be a fish out of water. Clearly I needed advice, and the man to give it was, obviously, William Castle.

The meeting with Castle was, as usual, entirely to the point. He had, he said, only one question: "Does the idea of going to the Children's Hospital make you happy?" When I told him that indeed it made me very happy, but also worried that I would fail, he made a classic comment: "Well, most people who come to see me are unhappy. You'd better go to Children's." I thought about that statement for a few moments and realized that he was completely correct.

The next day I accepted Dr. Janeway's offer, and a week or two later, in 1966, trundled my rudimentary laboratory equipment over the bridge to Children's to start a new life as an assistant professor of pediatrics. The laboratory in the basement of an about-to-be-constructed outpatient building was quite small and encumbered by a benchload of technicians who did the blood tests on research patients. My office was just large enough for a small desk and chair. A toilet tank on the wall flushed water into a plastic pipe. I worried vaguely about its symbolism. But the strength of the new surroundings was evident in the people. Dr. Diamond's fellows were waiting for their new boss expectantly. They were of the quality of Bill Mentzer, Eli Schwartz, and Bob Baehner. Steve Shohet came over with me from the Brigham, and soon Y. W. Kan, who had been a fellow with Frank Gardner, arrived from Philadelphia. That was the starting team, and it was a powerful one. Soon we were focused on thalassemia and the congenital hemolytic anemias. We even launched into granulocyte metabolism when we discovered the basis of the microbicidal defect in chronic granulomatous disease. Fifteen years later Stuart Orkin cloned the gene which, when mutated, causes most of the cases of that disease.

Though we were crammed into a very small space, I remained convinced that we could grow the new division if we attracted bright fellows, attacked important problems of high clinical relevance, and maintained high standards of technical training. Physician-scientists have a deadly tendency: they tend to learn a laboratory technique and then apply it as broadly as possible rather than asking new tough questions the solutions to which require new technology. Later Joe Goldstein called that sad state PAIDS (Paralyzed Academic Investigator's Disease Syndrome) (Goldstein 1986).

To fight off PAIDS, we encouraged our trainees to seek experience in basic laboratories at Harvard and MIT and at Harvard Medical School. We also recruited new fellows from a broad base of the very best internists and pediatricians, many from the fine Children's Hospital house staff training program. Some, like Arthur Nienhuis and Frank Bunn, came for only a year or two. Others, such as Bernie Forget, Sam Lux, Stuart Orkin, Y. W. Kan, and Tom Stossel, stayed much longer. Lux and Orkin ultimately assumed the leadership of the division. Still others such as Herb Abelson and Harvey Cohen became chairs of departments of pediatrics across the country. As we became better known, excellent candidates applied from abroad and returned to their countries to assume leadership positions.

Between 1966 and 1985 the division grew steadily in space, responsibilities, and people. In 1974 a collaboration with Emil Frei, the new president of the Dana-Farber Cancer Institute, produced a joint division of pediatric hematology and oncology co-sponsored by Children's Hospital and Dana-Farber. Hematology, including inpatient marrow transplantation, became the responsibility of Children's, while oncology leadership was assumed by Dana-Farber. All of the inpatient beds remained at Children's. That infusion of resources greatly expanded our training capacity.

By the time I left the leadership of the division in 1985, the combined division had risen to world-class status. Nine of the trainees became members of the National Academies, eight joined the Howard Hughes Medical Institute, four became fellows of the American Academy of Arts and Sciences, one became a member of the American Philosophical Society, thirty were elected to the Association of American Physicians, fifty-two were elected to the American Society for Clinical Investigation, thirty-six became members of the American Pediatric Society, and sixty-two were elected to the Society of Pediatric Research. Five presidents of the American Society for Clinical Investigation and four presidents of the American Society of Hematology were or had been members of the program. We trained scores of professors, deans, institute directors, and even a college president.

During the next two decades my own research interests embraced several areas. Most of my effort was still directed toward the pathophysiology and treatment of thalassemia. In 1970 I spent a very important sabbatical in the biology department at MIT in the laboratory shared by Harvey Lodish and David Baltimore. Under Harvey's expert direction I examined the translation of thalassemic beta globin messenger RNA and found that the message that made contact with ribosomes behaved normally. Therefore we concluded that the root cause of the disease must be low production of beta globin message.

That conclusion was reasonable but turned out later to be incomplete. Many beta thalassemia mutations do affect the function as well as the content of beta globin message. In the same year Baltimore isolated reverse transcriptase, a discovery that earned him a Nobel Prize. This new reagent, coupled with Hamilton Smith's and the late Dan Nathans's Nobel Prize–winning discovery of restriction enzymes completely changed thalassemia research. Edward Benz, then a student in the lab, worked with Bernie Forget and members of the Lodish-Baltimore lab to prove without doubt that beta thalassemia is due to either low production or low function of beta globin messenger RNA (Housman et al. 1979). A few years later Stuart Orkin demonstrated many of the point mutations in and deletions of the beta and alpha globin genes that characterize the disease (Kazazian et al. 1984). Y. W. Kan, who moved with Steve Shohet to the University of California, San Francisco, made many important molecular discoveries as well (Chang et al. 1979). In fact Kan is rightly considered a father of molecular medicine.

Although the new molecular genetics fascinated me, I wanted to focus my efforts on treatment and prevention. In the 1970s Susan Shurin, Richard Propper, and I decided to attack iron overload, the most lethal consequence of the transfusion management of thalassemia. We started with continuous intravenous deferoxamine and then, as a practical alternative, devised continuous subcutaneous administration of the drug via the first portable infusion pump, made in a basement in Brooklyn by Dean Kamen. The method worked and saved countless lives, but it was not at all well accepted by teenagers, and many patients developed painful welts at the sites of injections. Almost thirty years later I was able to contribute to the development of deferasirox, an orally active iron chelator with a very long dwell time in the blood. I am hopeful that the drug may replace deferoxamine.

While Y. W. Kan, Blanche Alter, and Henry Chang were with me at Children's, we approached the problem of prenatal diagnosis of thalassemia and sickle cell disease. In the midst of our work, Kan moved to California and continued the research there. He was actually the first to perform a successful prenatal diagnosis using fetal blood (Kan et al. 1975). We worked with Bernadette Modell and Ernie Huehns in London and with John Hobbins and Maurice Mahoney at Yale to employ the fetoscope to obtain the fetal blood samples. Shortly thereafter Stuart Orkin joined us, and we became the first team to utilize cDNA probes of fetal fibroblast DNA to rule out the diagnosis of beta thalassemia in a fetus at risk. The fetal blood and DNA approaches were almost immediately adopted by Antonio Cao in Sardinia (Cao et al. 1984) and by Dimitris Loukopoulos in Greece (Loukopoulos, Kaltysoya-Tassiopoulou, and Fessas 1988). Their efforts greatly reduced the births of neonates with severe thalassemia. Our employment of the fetoscope was strongly opposed by "Right to Life" partisans (Nathan 1974), but the work in Europe went on unabated. Thalassemia can be prevented, and in my opinion prevention is surely the most reasonable and cost-effective way to reduce the impact of the disease.

I summarized much of my experience of thalassemia in a book published in 1995 about the course of one patient, titled *Genes, Blood, and Courage* (Nathan 1995). Those were exciting days of advancing technology and rapid translation of that technology to patients and their families. Those brave patients served as the experimental models—many of them knowing that only others would be the beneficiaries. I remain in awe of them.

By the mid-1970s I had established a new oncology-based laboratory at Dana-Farber and felt that the focus of my efforts should be on areas of greater relevance to the cancer patient. Returning to my initial interest in the regulation of erythropoiesis, I took another sabbatical with David Housman at MIT to learn more about measurements of in vitro hematopoiesis. This helped me contribute to further understanding of Diamond Blackfan anemia, and to grasp that human in vitro erythropoiesis requires, in addition to erythropoietin, other kinase activators produced by marrow adventitial cells and T cells.

Just before I entered the Housman laboratory, Brian Clarke, one of Housman's postdoctoral fellows, had shown that some of the colonies of human red cells derived from progenitors in vitro express substantial quantities of fetal hemoglobin, reminding me of the fetal-like "stress" erythropoiesis observed in marrow failure or hemolytic anemia. When I returned to my laboratory at Dana-Farber, I took on that problem. Joined by Barbara Miller, I examined the unusual patients with sickle cell anemia who live and work in the hot eastern oases of Saudi Arabia. They have relatively few symptoms because their red cells contain up to 30 percent fetal hemoglobin. Saudi patients with sickle trait have normal levels of fetal hemoglobin, but their progenitor-derived erythroid colonies make vast amounts. Clearly the hemolytic stress of sickle cell anemia stimulates the hemoglobin F expression. Joined by Stuart Orkin, we showed that these patients have a mutation in one of the two promoters of fetal hemoglobin structural genes. Today Vijay Sankaran, a Harvard MD-PhD student in Orkin's laboratory, is working on that problem in much greater detail (Lettre et al. 2008).

The benefit of fetal hemoglobin in sickle cell anemia patients made me wonder whether drugs that stimulate rapid erythropoiesis might be useful in American patients with sickle cell anemia. The work of

Joseph DeSimone and Paul Heller in Chicago and Tim Ley and Arthur Nienhuis at NIH greatly influenced my thinking. DeSimone and Heller gave 5-azacytidine, a drug that is an S phase inhibitor and an inhibitor of DNA methylation, to bled baboons. They observed a vast increase in fetal hemoglobin over baseline. Ley and Nienhuis had the courage to give the drug to patients with thalassemia. There was a clear increase in fetal hemoglobin in those patients, and Ley and Nienhuis posited that the fetal hemoglobin promoters might have become demethylated and hence more active. My former student Edward J. Benz Jr., then at Yale, wrote a stirring editorial in the *New England Journal of Medicine* in which he opined that molecular biology had come to the bedside (Benz 1982), but I wasn't at all sure. I thought the S phase inhibition induced by 5-azacytidine had transiently depressed erythropoiesis in the baboons and the patients. As their erythropoiesis recovered, the "stress" was reflected by increased fetal hemoglobin synthesis just as we had observed in the Saudi patients.

But how should this hypothesis be tested? Hydroxyurea is an S phase inhibitor, but it has no known effect on DNA epigenetics. Why not give sickle cell anemia patients hydroxyurea and observe their fetal hemoglobin responses? When I proposed this, I ran into a brick wall. Neither Orah Platt, who was at that time in charge of the sickle cell anemia clinic, nor Stuart Orkin, who had become the leader of our hemoglobin research program, would have anything to do with the idea unless I could demonstrate that hydroxyurea works in a simian model. Fortunately Norman Letvin, an experimental immunologist interested in AIDS, maintained a colony of cynmologous monkeys at the New England Primate Center. He collaborated with our team, and we showed that hydroxyurea stimulates fetal hemoglobin accumulation in the red cells of these monkeys when they are rendered anemic by bleeding. With that information in hand, Orah Platt gave the drug to two patients with sickle cell anemia. Both responded, and hydroxyurea became the first drug to modify the clinical course of the disease.

In 1985 I became the physician in chief and chief of the Department of Medicine at Children's Hospital. These were the posts held by Charles A. Janeway when he brought me to the department in 1966. It was an honor to sit in that office and try to emulate what Janeway had brought to academic pediatrics. Janeway's photograph and those of William Castle and Samuel A. Levine were always close at hand to remind me of what quality leadership could be. Steven Burakoff and Sam Lux directed the hematology-oncology division and worked together to maintain the clinical care, the training program, and the research. A laboratory which included Colin Sieff and Bernard Mathey-Prevot and myself continued to explore the interstices of in vitro hematopoiesis, assisted by a productive relationship with Steven Clark and the Genetics Institute.

Just as the ten-year term in the department to which I had committed was coming to an end, a crisis occurred at Dana-Farber involving an overdose of chemotherapy. The leading trustees asked me to take over and address the problem, which I did in 1995. Though I was finally forced to give up my laboratory because of time pressures, I was indeed fortunate in that position. The staff and the trustees pulled together to create important collaborations within the Harvard Medical School. The results were productive clinical programs, including Dana-Farber–Children's Hospital Cancer Care and Dana-Farber–Brigham and Women's Hospital Cancer Care. The development of the Dana-Farber–Harvard Cancer Center provided an opportunity for a research collaboration that united all of the Harvard health institutions in cancer research. A new research building allowed Dana-Farber to recruit new investigators with marvelous credentials. I describe some of the advances in oncology in my book *The Cancer Treatment Revolution* (Nathan 2007a). During that five-year period I also chaired the Director's Panel on Clinical Research for Harold Varmus, then the director of NIH. Our panel came up with recommendations for new grants to support clinical research which have made a substantial difference in the lives of those who aspire to succeed in the field. And private charities such as the Doris Duke Charitable Trust, the Burroughs Wellcome Foundation, and the Howard Hughes Medical Institute have developed unique supporting programs for clinical investigators.

Toward the end of my five-year term in 2000 a wonderful event occurred. Thanks to the generosity of many, especially Dana-Farber trustees Stephen Swensrud and the late Anne E Dyson, MD, Harvard Medical School established the David G. Nathan Chair in Pediatric Hematology and Oncology. The first incumbent is Stuart Orkin, who became my chief as I settled back into the division. My replacement as Dana-Farber president is my former great student Edward J. Benz Jr. What could be a better coda to a life in academic medicine? I have been honored to receive many very prestigious awards and memberships in distinguished societies. They include the Howland Medal of the American Pediatric Society (Lovejoy 2004; Nathan 2004) and the Kober Medal of the Association of American Physicians (Benz 2007; Nathan 2007b). The bibliographies in the papers that celebrate those awards contain references to most of the research efforts described here. But that chair and the fact that my chiefs are my own former trainees are the highest rewards of all. They make me realize once again that Dr. Castle was correct. A focus on the patient can lead to an exhilarating and successful career in academic medicine. I am so deeply fortunate to have had mentors who guided me toward that path.

Epilogue

LOOKING FORWARD

Andrew I. Schafer, MD

The central premise of this work has been that physicians, working as active researchers, have throughout history played, and must in the future continue to play, a vital role in the advancement of medical knowledge. Informed by their personal experiences in caring for patients, they are irreplaceably positioned at the interface between fundamental biomedical science and clinical practice. Yet today a convergence of transformational forces threatens the future viability of physician-scientists, at least in the form in which we currently recognize them. As described in the foregoing chapters, these forces are a combination of social, cultural, educational, demographic, ecological, and economic in nature. Failure of our academic institutions and research funding agencies to recognize them and respond to them proactively places our society at risk of squandering its most outstanding intellectual talent in populating the workforce of physician-scientists for generations to come.

The breathtaking pace and scope of progress in both the science and practice of medicine during this generation have vastly outstripped the capacity of any individual physician-scientist to maintain even the semblance of currency in both arenas. By necessity, medical research has become a "team sport." It has become impossible for medical schools, or even combined MD-PhD programs, to impart anything more than the rudiments of these bodies of knowledge to their students. What is taught often becomes rapidly outdated or even obsolete. Furthermore, there is serious concern that medical schools and postgraduate clinical training programs are increasingly deemphasizing the scientific basis of medical practice. The teaching of diagnosis and treatment of disease is increasingly becoming evidence-based. While this is a laudable development, it cannot be confused with or replace pathophysiology-based medical education.

The landmasses of basic biomedical research and clinical practice, which the great physician-scientists of the twentieth century could navigate with such facility, have progressively separated. The widening chasm between them has even created a language barrier between basic scientists and clinicians. It has spawned the formal recognition of "translational" medicine as a critical link, albeit much more easily described as a catchphrase than effectively executed in practice. While acknowledging that there is strong disagreement about this point, even among some authors of this volume, I believe that the recent movement to make translational medicine a distinct "discipline" may be misguided. Rather than attempting to separate it, we should view it as the very core of all medical research.

With the growth of an enormous workforce of highly specialized PhD biomedical scientists, physicians engaged in basic research have found themselves having to retreat increasingly into their laboratories to remain competitive with their PhD colleagues. The resultant disappearance of serious physician-scientists from the hospital wards and clinics has made them largely invisible as potential role models to medical trainees who might be interested in research careers. At the same time, important demographic and cultural changes have begun to impact profoundly the choice of research careers of medical school graduates. The extraordinary intellectual powerbase of women as the future majority of physicians will be lost if they continue to find academic medical research careers as inhospitable as they do today. The next generations of medical school graduates, irrespective of gender, will place greater importance on work-life balance and controllable lifestyles, characteristics that previous generations of physician-scientists have considered incompatible with a serious career commitment to research.

Finally, the increasing unpredictability of governmental support for medical research is driving the most brilliant potential young physician-scientists away from research and into more secure career paths in clinical practice. Major economic downturns, as experienced worldwide at the time of this writing, pose a particularly great risk to sustaining continuity in the medical research workforce if its funding is allowed to become too dependent on limited sources (e.g., the NIH). Only a strong and stable balance of support from the government, foundations, industry, philanthropy, and institutional endowments, coordinated through partnerships among these sponsor entities, can provide assurance to the next generation that medical research is a viable and durable career opportunity.

Not all of these forces should be viewed purely as threats to the future of physician-scientists. Indeed many of them could be creatively parlayed to its advantage. Throughout history the physician-scientist "species" has repeatedly faced greater perils than those that exist today, including world wars, economic catastrophes, and monumental upheavals in the delivery and financing of health care. Yet physician-scientists have always succeeded in reinventing themselves by not only adapting to the times but also actually forging many of the revolutionary changes that have allowed them to flourish.

What, then, might the next generation of physician-scientists look like? First, the pipeline will, by design, originate at earlier, more formative stages of education. Strong and durable bridges will have been built to foster their career path, spanning high school, university, medical school, graduate medical education, and initial faculty appointments. Continuity will be secured through funded linkages among these currently separated phases of development. Accommodations for fast-tracking across these stages will permit entry into independent research careers at a considerably younger age than is the case today for many individuals.

Just as "moving up" and "stepping off" have been the only options available to other workers on the traditional corporate ladder since the industrial revolution, "up or out" has been the rigidly binary system of promotion and tenure for physician-scientist faculty of medical schools for much of the past century. But now institutions must confront the reality that emerging generations will increasingly reject the life tradeoffs required by a winner-take-all mentality in academic medicine. Token attempts by medical schools to extend the promotion and tenure "clocks" for fixed and very limited periods to allow women (and men) time for early child care will be simply inadequate. Those academic medical centers that can make a substantive commitment to recognizing and embracing individualized and personalized paces and patterns of career growth will quickly find themselves at a distinct competitive advantage in recruiting and retaining the best physician-scientist minds. So, after an inevitable period of resistance from an ivory tower that was built for a workforce of earlier times, physician-scientist faculty will be liberated from the anachronistic promotion and tenure rules of today's academe. The current misalignment between the traditional workplace and a largely nontraditional workforce (Benko and Weisberg 2007) will be reconciled. Fluid, dynamic, and customized career trajectories will be accommodated, including "off-ramps" and "on-ramps" to full-time employment, as well as some control over hours, pace, and workload (with commensurate modulation of compensation and position) to balance career and life demands. A new culture of personalized career design for future generations of physician-scientists will certainly continue to accommodate and reward the many who will choose a life of sustained, intense immersion in the work of academic medicine. The continued maturation of team science, with opportunities for individuals to assume different and changing roles in the research teams (as illustrated in figure 0.2 in the introduction), should fit well into the customized career paths of tomorrow.

In striking contrast to the situation that existed as recently as two or three decades ago, there is currently a disproportionate decline among young physician-scientists who are interested in basic science (as opposed to clinical) research. At least as far as this may be due to their increasing disadvantage in competing with PhD investigators who can devote their nearly full attention to fundamental science, the emergence of team research should help reverse the swing of the pendulum and bring many physicians back into the laboratory. At the same time, PhD scientists should feel increasingly comfortable in the clinical research arena as they receive more direct exposure to clinical medicine during their training.

This hopeful landscape of tomorrow promises to narrow today's chasm between the landmasses of basic biomedical research and clinical practice. Physician-scientists should be considered "endangered" today only in their current state, not in the sense of permanent extinction. They must not and will not vanish. Indeed, their future can be as bright as ever if we proactively fashion it with creativity, foresight, and vision.

References

Adler RE. 2004. *Medical Firsts: From Hippocrates to the Human Genome*. Hoboken, NJ: John Wiley & Sons.

Ahn J, Watt CD, Man L-X, Greeley SA, Shea JA. 2007. Educating future leaders of medical research: analysis of student opinions and goals from the MD-PhD SAGE (Students' Attitudes, Goals, and Education) Survey. Acad. Med. 82:633–45.

Ahrens EH Jr. 1992. *The Crisis in Clinical Research: Overcoming Institutional Obstacles*. New York: Oxford University Press.

Aisenberg N, Harrington M. 1988. *Women of Academe: Outsiders in the Sacred Grove*. Amherst: University of Massachusetts Press.

Altman LK. 1998. *Who Goes First?* Berkeley: University of California Press.

Amazigo U, Noma M, Bump J, et al. 2006. Onchocerciasis. In Jamison DT, Feachem RG, Makgoba MW et al., eds., *Disease and Mortality in Sub-Saharan Africa*. Washington, DC: World Bank Publications. 215–22.

Anderson MS, Horn AS, Risbey KR. 2007. What do mentoring and training in the responsible conduct of research have to do with scientists' misbehaviors? Findings from a national survey of NIH funded scientists. Acad. Med. 82:853–60.

Andrews N. 2007. Climbing through medicine's glass ceiling. N. Engl. J. Med. 357: 1887.

Andrews NC. 2002. The other physician-scientist problem: where have all the young girls gone? Nat. Med. 8:439–41.

Antman EM, Giugliano RP, Gibson CM, et al. 1999. Abciximab facilitates the rate and extent of thrombolysis: results of the thrombolysis in myocardial infarction (TIMI) 14 trial. The TIMI 14 Investigators. Circulation 99:2720–32.

Archer SL. 2007. The making of a physician-scientist—the process has a pattern: lessons from the lives of Nobel laureates in medicine and physiology. Eur. Heart J. 28(4):510–14.

Arias IM. 1989. Training basic scientists to bridge the gap between basic science and its application to human disease. N. Engl. J. Med. 321:972–74.

Aschwanden C. 2008. Managing to excel at science. Cell 132:911–13.

Association of American Medical Colleges. 2000a. *For the Health of the Public: Ensuring the Future of Clinical Research.* Volume 1. Report of the AAMC Task Force on Clinical Research. Ralph Snyderman, MD, chair. Washington, DC: AAMC.

Association of American Medical Colleges. 2000b. Medical Schools Objectives Project. *Contemporary Issues in Medicine: Basic Science and Clinical Research.* Report 4. Dennis Ausiello, MD, chair, clinical research panel. Washington, DC: AAMC. Available at http://www.med.mun.ca/ugme/docs/msop4.pdf, accessed Oct. 23, 2008.

Association of American Medical Colleges. 2002a. *Information Technology Enabling Clinical Research.* Washington, DC: AAMC.

Association of American Medical Colleges. 2002b. *Protecting Subjects, Preserving Trust, Promoting Progress II.* Report of the Task Force on Financial Conflicts of Interest in Human Subjects Research. Washington, DC: AAMC. Available at http://www.aamc.org/research/coi/2002coireport.pdf, accessed Oct. 23, 2008.

Association of American Medical Colleges. 2006a. *Statement on the Physician Workforce.* Available at http://www.aamc.org/workforce/workforceposition.pdf, accessed Sept. 10, 2008.

Association of American Medical Colleges. 2006b. *Promoting Translational and Clinical Science: The Critical Role of Medical Schools and Teaching Hospitals.* Report of the AAMC's Task Force II on Clinical Research. Steven G. Gabbe, MD, chair. Washington, DC: AAMC. Available at http://www.aamc.org/promotingclinicalscience, accessed Oct. 23, 2008.

Association of American Medical Colleges. 2008a. *GQ All Schools Report.* Available at http://www.aamc.org/data/gq/allschoolsreports/start.htm, accessed Aug. 19, 2008.

Association of American Medical Colleges. 2008b. Women in Medicine (website). Available at http://www.aamc.org/members/wim/, accessed March 26, 2008.

Association of American Medical Colleges and the American Medical Association. 1999. *Clinical Research: A National Call to Action. Graylyn.* Washington, DC: AAMC.

Association of American Medical Colleges and the American Medical Association. 1998. National Clinical Research Summit Project: *Graylyn Conference Report.* Washington, DC: AAMC.

Association of American Medical Colleges and the American Medical Association. 1999. *Clinical Research: A National Call to Action.* Washington, DC: AAMC.

Association of American Medical Colleges and the Association of American Universities. 2008. *Protecting Patients, Preserving Integrity, Advancing Health: Accelerating the Implementation of COI Policies in Human Subjects Research.* Report of the AAMC-AAU Advisory Committee on Financial Conflicts of Interest in Human Subjects Research. Robert R. Rich, MD, Mark S. Wrighton, MD, co-chairs. Washington, DC: AAMC. Available at https://services.aamc.org/Publications/showfile.cfm?file=version107.pdf&prd_id=220&prv_id=268&pdf_id=107, accessed Oct. 23, 2008.

Atchley DW. 1961. *Physician: Healer and Scientist.* New York: Macmillan.

Baer I, Feiler ME, Regulski A, Switzer SS. 2004. *Clinical Trial Contracts: A Discussion of Four Selected Provisions.* Washington, DC: AAMC. Available at https://services.aamc.org/Publications/showfile.cfm?file=version6.pdf&prd_id=76&prv_id=75&pdf_id=6, accessed Oct. 22, 2008.

Balistreri WF, Jobe A, Boat TF. 2006. Pediatric subspecialty training fellowships at Cincinnati Children's Hospital Medical Center. J. Pediatr. 147:277–78.

Banting F. 1965. *Nobel Lectures, Physiology or Medicine, 1922–1941.* Amsterdam: Elsevier.

Barzansky B, Etzel SI. 2003. Medical schools in the United States, 2002–2003. JAMA 290:1190–96.

Barzansky B, Etzel SI. 2005. Medical schools in the United States, 2004–2005. JAMA 294:1068–74.

Baskett TF. 2002. The resuscitation greats: William O'Shaughnessy, Thomas Latta, and the origins of intravenous saline. Resuscitation 55:231–34.

Baughman KL, Duffy FD, Eagle KA, Faxon DP, Hillis LD, Lange RA. 2008. Task force 1: training in clinical cardiology. J. Am. Coll. Cardiol. 51(3):339–48.

Benko C, Weisberg A. 2007. *Mass Career Customization: Aligning the Workplace with Today's Nontraditional Workforce.* Boston: Harvard Business School Press.

Benz EJ. 1982. Clinical management of gene expression. N. Engl. J. Med. 307: 1515–16.

Benz EJ. 2007. Association of American Physicians George M. Kober Medal: introduction of David G. Nathan, MD. J. Clin. Invest. 117:1107–11.

Bernard C. 1927. *An Introduction to the Study of Experimental Medicine.* New York: Macmillan.

Bickel J, Brown AJ. 2005. Generation X: Implications for faculty recruitment and development at academic health centers. Acad. Med. 80:205–10.

Bickel J, Wara D, Atkinson B, et al. 2002. Increasing women's leadership in academic medicine: report of the AAMC Project Implementation Committee. Acad. Med. 77(10):1043–61.

Bland CJ, Schmitz CC. 1986. Characteristics of the successful researcher and implications for faculty development. J. Med. Educ. 61:22–31.

Bliss M. 1999. *William Osler: A Life in Medicine.* Toronto: University of Toronto Press.

Blue R, Murcia M, Karan C, Jirouskova M, Coller BS. 2008. Application of high throughput screening to identify a novel αIIb-specific small molecule inhibitor of αIIbβ3-mediated platelet interaction with fibrinogen. Blood 111:1248–56.

Bond E, Butler WT, Gallin ET, Pardue M-L, Pion G, Sechrest L, Hollingsworth Smith L, Weldon VW, Wyngaarden JB. 2004. *Bridging the Bed-Bench Gap: Contributions of the Markey Trust.* Washington, DC: National Academies Press. Bowles MD, Dawson VP. 2003. *With One Voice: The Association of American Medical Colleges, 1876–2002.* Washington, DC: AAMC.

Brown AJ, Friedman AH. 2007. Challenges and opportunities for recruiting a new generation of neurosurgeons. Neurosurgery 61:1314–21.

Brown AJ, Swinyard W, Ogle J. 2003. Women in academic medicine: a report of focus groups and questionnaires, with conjoint analysis. J. Women's Health 12:999.

Buckley LM, Sanders K, Shih M, et al. 2000. Obstacles to promotion? Values of women faculty about career success and recognition. Acad. Med. 75(3):283–88.

Bunn HF. 2007. Castle and Jandl: Pioneers of experimental hematology. Hematologist 4(5).

Butler D. 2008. Translational research: crossing the valley of death. Nature 453:840–42.

Bynum WF, Hardy A, Jacyna S, Lawrence C, Tansey EM. 2006. The Western Medical Tradition, 1800 to 2000. Cambridge: Cambridge University Press.

Campbell EG, Weissman JS, Blumenthal D. 1997. Relationship between market competition and the activities and attitudes of medical school faculty. JAMA 278(3):222–26.

Cao A, Pintus L, Lecca U, Olla G, Cossu P, Rosatelli C, Galanello R. 1984. Control of homozygous beta-thalassemia by carrier screening and antenatal diagnosis in Sardinians. Clin. Genet. 26:12–22.

Carr P, Ash AS, Friedman R, et al. 1998. Relation of family responsibilities and gender to productivity and career satisfaction of medical faculty. Ann. Intern. Med. 129(7):532–38.

Carr PL, Ash AS, Friedman RH, et al. 2000. Faculty perceptions of gender discrimination and sexual harassment in academic medicine. Ann. Intern. Med. 132(11):889–96.

Chang JC, Temple GF, Trecartin RF, Kan YW. 1979. Suppression of the nonsense mutation in homozygous beta 0 thalassaemia. Nature 281:602–3.

Clough JD. 2004. *To Act as a Unit: The Story of the Cleveland Clinic.* 4th ed. Cleveland: Cleveland Clinic Press.

Cole R. 1920. The university department of medicine. Science 51:329–40.

Cole R. 1926. The modern hospital and medical progress. Science 64:123–30.

Cole R. 1949. Dr. Osler: scientist and teacher. Arch. Intern. Med. 84:54–63.

Coller BS. 1980. Interaction of normal, thrombasthenic, and Bernard-Soulier platelets with immobilized fibrinogen: defective platelet-fibrinogen interaction in thrombasthenia. Blood 55:169–78.

Coller BS. 1985. A new murine monoclonal antibody reports an activation-dependent change in the conformation and/or microenvironment of the platelet GPIIb/IIIa complex. J. Clin. Invest. 76:101–8.

Coller BS. 1995. Blockade of platelet GPIIb/IIIa receptors as an antithrombotic strategy. Circulation 92:2373–80.

Coller BS. 1998. Monitoring platelet GPIIb/IIIa antagonist therapy. Circulation 97:5–9.

Coller BS. 2006. The physician-scientist, the state, and the oath: thoughts for our times. J. Clin. Invest. 116:2567–70.

Coller BS, Anderson K, Weisman HF. 1995. Inhibitors of platelet aggregation: GPIIb/IIIa Antagonists. In Braunwald E, ed., *Heart Disease: A Textbook of Cardiovascular Medicine*, Update 4. Philadelphia: W. B. Saunders. 1–10.

Coller BS, Klotman P, Smith LG. 2002. Professing and living the oath: teaching medicine as a profession. Am. J. Med. 112:744–48.

Coller BS, Peerschke EI, Scudder LE, Sullivan CA. 1983. A murine monoclonal antibody that completely blocks the binding of fibrinogen to platelets produces a thrombasthenic-like state in normal platelets and binds to glycoproteins IIb and/or IIIa. J. Clin. Invest. 72:325–38.

Collins-Nakai R. 2006. Leadership in medicine. McGill J. Med. 9:68–73.

Committee on Maximizing the Potential of Women in Academic Science and Engineering, National Academy of Sciences, National Academy of Engineering, and Institute of Medicine. 2006. *Beyond Bias and Barriers: Fulfilling the Potential of Women in Academic Science and Engineering.* Washington, DC: National Academies Press.

Conti F. 2001. Claude Bernard: primer of the second biomedical revolution. Nature Rev. 2:703–8.

Cornett D. 2005. Expectations of Gen-X recruitment candidates. Physician's News Digest January, http://www.physiciansnews.com/expectations-of-gen-x-recruitment-candidates/.

Council of Graduate Schools. 1995. *A Conversation about Mentoring: Trends and Models.* Washington, DC: Council of Graduate Schools.

Council NR, ed. 2005. *Bridges to Independence: Fostering the Independence of New Investigators in Biomedical Research.* Washington, DC: National Academies Press. 34–73.

Davies K, White M. 1995. *Breakthrough: The Race to Find the Breast Cancer Gene.* New York: John Wiley and Sons.

De Angelis CD, Johns ME. 1995. Promotion of women in academic medicine: shatter the ceilings, polish the floors. JAMA 273(13):1056–57.

De Angelis C, Drazen JM, Frizelle FA, Haug C, Hoey J, Horton R, et al. Clinical trial registration: a statement from the International Committee of Medical Journal Editors. Ann Intern Med. 2004;141:477–78.

De Angelis C, Drazen JM, Frizelle FA, Haug C, Hoey J, Horton R, et al. Is this clinical trial fully registered? A statement from the International Committee of Medical Journal Editors. NEJM 2005; 352(23):2436–438.

Dickler HB, Fang D, Heinig SJ, Johnson E, Korn D. 2007. New physician-investigators receiving National Institutes of Health research project grants: a historical perspective on the "endangered species." JAMA 297(22):2496–2501.

Dickler HB, Korn D, Gabbe SG. 2006. Promoting translational and clinical science: the critical role of medical schools and teaching hospitals. PLoS Medicine 3(9):e378.

Donowitz M, Germino G, Cominelli F, Anderson JM. 2007. The attrition of young physician-scientists: problems and potential solutions. Gastroenterology 132:477–80.

Dorsey ER, Jarjoura D, Rutecki GW. 2003. Influence of controllable lifestyle on recent trends in specialty choice by US medical students. JAMA 290:1173–78.

Dorsey ER, Jarjoura D, Rutecki GW. 2005. The influence of controllable lifestyle and sex on the specialty choices of graduating US medical students, 1996–2003. Acad. Med. 80(9):791–96.

Dubos RJ. 1976. *The Professor, the Institute, and DNA*. New York: Rockefeller University Press.

Ehringhaus S, Korn D. 2002. Conflicts of interest in human subjects research. Issues in Science and Technology Winter.

Ehringhaus S, Korn D. 2006. Principles for protecting integrity in the conduct and reporting of clinical trials. A white paper. Association of American Medical Colleges. Available at http://www.aamc.org/research/clinicaltrialsreporting/clinical trialsreporting.pdf, accessed Oct. 21, 2008.

Eichna LW. 1972. Presentation of the Academy Medal to James A. Shannon, MD. Bull. NY Acad. Med. 48:1194–98.

Elrod, JM, Karnad, AB. 2003. Boston City Hospital and the Thorndike Memorial Laboratory: the birth of modern haematology. Br. J. Haematol. 121:383–89.

Emans SJ, Goldberg CT, Milstein ME, Dobriner J. 2008. Creating a faculty development office in an academic pediatric hospital: challenges and successes. Pediatrics 390–401.

EPIC Investigators. 1994. Use of a monoclonal antibody directed against the platelet glycoprotein IIb/IIIa receptor in high-risk coronary angioplasty. N. Engl. J. Med. 330:956–61.

Epps RP, Bernstein AE. 1990. Day care programs affiliated with teaching hospitals: report of the Dependent Care Task Force. J. Am. Med. Women's Assoc. 45(1):20–22.

Fang D, Dickler HB, Heinig SJ, Korn D. 2007. *Recruitment of New Physician Investigators in Clinical Research: Finding from a Survey of Clinical Department Chairs at US Medical Schools*. Monograph. Washington, DC: AAMC. Available at https://services.aamc. org/Publications/index.cfm?fuseaction=Product.displayForm&prd_id=211&prv_ id=255, accessed Oct. 23, 2008.

Fang D, Meyer RE. 2003. PhD faculty in clinical departments of US medical schools, 1981–1999: their widening presence and roles in research. Academic Medicine 78(12):1271–80.

Fangerau HM. 2006. The novel *Arrowsmith*, Paul de Kruif (1890–1971), and Jacques Loeb (1859–1924): a literary portrait of "medical science." Medical Humanities (an edition of the Journal for Medical Ethics) 32:82–87.

Feinstein AR. 1999. Basic biomedical science and the destruction of the pathophysiologic bridge from bench to bedside. Am. J. Med. 107:461–67.

Ferry G. 2007. *Max Perutz and the Secret of Life*. Woodbury, NY: Cold Spring Harbor Laboratory Press.

Fisher K, Mays D. 2008. *AAMC Teaching Hospitals and Health Systems: Serving the Nation through Education, Research, and Patient Care*. Washington, DC: AAMC.

Food and Drug Administration. 2000. PL 106–505, sections 201–207, enacted November 2000.

Food and Drug Administration. 2007. PL 110–85, Food and Drug Administration Amendments Act of 2007.

French DL, Coller BS, Berkowitz R, et al. 1998. Prenatal diagnosis of Glanzmann thrombasthenia using the polymorphic markers BRCA 1 and THRA 1 on chromosome 17. Br. J. Haematol. 102:582–87.

Fried LP, Francomano CA, MacDonald SM, et al. 1996. Career development for women in academic medicine: multiple interventions in a department of medicine. JAMA 276(11):898–905.

Froom JD, Bickel J. 1996. Medical school policies for part-time faculty committed to full professional effort. Acad. Med. 71(1):91–96.

Gairdner WT. 1889. *The Physician as Naturalist: Addresses and Memoirs Bearing on the History and Progress of Medicine*. Glasgow: James Maclehose & Sons.

Gale, SF. 2007. Bridging the gap. PM Network. March:26–31.

Giancola F. 2006. The generation gap: more myth than reality. Human Resource Planning 29:32–37.

Gill GN. 1984. The end of the physician-scientist? Am. Scholar 53:353–69.

Ginsburg GS, Burke TW, Febbo P. 2008. Centralized bio-repositories for genetic and genomoic research. JAMA 299:1359–61.

Gitterman DP, Greenwood RS, Kocis KC, Mayes BR, McKethan AN. 2004. Did a rising tide lift all boats? The NIH budget and pediatric research portfolio. Health. Aff. (Millwood) 23:113–24.

Gold HK, Gimple L, Yasuda T, et al. 1990. Pharmacodynamic study of F(ab')2 fragments of murine monoclonal antibody 7E3 directed against human platelet glycoprotein IIb/IIIa, in patients with unstable angina pectoris. J. Clin. Invest. 86:651–59.

Goldstein J. 1986. On the origin and prevention of PAIDS (paralyzed academic investigator's disease syndrome). Presidential address delivered before the 78th Annual Meeting of the American Society for Clinical Investigation. J. Clin. Invest. 78:848–54.

Goldstein J. 2008. As doctors get a life, strains show. Wall Street Journal, April 29.

Goldstein J, Brown MS. 1997. The clinical investigator: bewitched, bothered, and bewildered—but still beloved. J. Clin. Invest. 99:2803–12.

Grande F, Visscher MB, eds. 1967. *Claude Bernard and Experimental Medicine*. Cambridge: Schenkman Publishing Company.

Gray ML, Bonventre JV. 2002. Training PhD researchers to translate science to clinical medicine: closing the gap from the other side. Nat. Med. 8:902–3.

Guelich JM, Singer BH, Castro MC, Rosenberg LE. 2002. A gender gap in the next generation of physician-scientists: medical student interest and participation in research. J. Investig. Med. 50:412–18.

Gunsalus CK, Bruner EM, Burbules NC. 2006. Mission creep in the IRB world. Science 312:1441.

Hamel MB, Ingelfinger JR, Phimister E, Solomon CG. 2006. Women in academic medicine: progress and challenges. N. Engl. J. Med. 355(3):310–11.

Haspel RL. 2006. Physician-scientist training (letter to editor). JAMA 295:623.

Heinig SJ, Krakower JY, Dickler HB, Korn D. 2007. Sustaining the engine of US biomedical discovery. N. Engl. J. Med. 357(10):1042–47.

Heinig SJ, Quon AS, Meyer RE, Korn D. 1999. The changing landscape for clinical research. Academic Medicine 74:726–45.

Hellman H. 2001. *Great Feuds in Medicine*. New York: John Wiley & Sons.

Hostetter MK. 2002. Career development for physician-scientists: the model of the Pediatric Scientist Development Program. J. Pediatr. 140(2):143–44.

Housman D, Forget BG, Skoultchi A, Benz EJ Jr. 1979. Quantitative deficiency of chain-specific globin messenger ribonucleic acids in beta thalassaemia. Nature 281(5732):602–3.

Howe N, Strauss W. 2007 The next twenty years: how customer and workforce attitudes will evolve. Harvard Business Review July–August:41–52.

Huang AJ. 1999. Reinventing the physician-scientist in the new era of health care. JAMA 281:94.

Institute of Medicine Clinical Research Roundtable. 2001. *The Clinical Investigator Workforce: Clinical Research Roundtable Symposium I, II, and III.* Washington, DC: National Academy Press.

Jackson VA, Palepu A, Szalacha L, et al. 2003. "Having the right chemistry": a qualitative study of mentoring in academic medicine. Acad. Med. 78:328–34.

Jagsi R, Butterton JR, Starr R, Tarbell NJ. 2007. A targeted intervention for the career development of women in academic medicine. Arch. Intern. Med. 167:343–45.

Jagsi R, Guancial EA, Worobey CC, et al. 2006. The "gender gap" in authorship of academic literature: a thirty-five-year perspective. New. Engl. J. Med. 355:281–87.

Jagsi R, Tarbell NJ, Henault LE, Chang Y, Hylek EM. 2008. The representation of women on the editorial boards of major medical journals: a thirty-five-year perspective. Arch. Intern. Med. 168:544–48.

Jagsi R, Tarbell NJ, Weinstein DW. 2007. Becoming a doctor, starting a family: leaves of absence from graduate medical education. N. Engl. J. Med. 357(19):1889–91.

Jobe AH, Abramson JS, Batshaw M, Boxer LA, Lister G, McCabe E, Johnston R. 2002. Work Groups on Research, American Pediatric Society. Recruitment and development of academic pediatricians: departmental commitments to promote success. Pediatr. Res. 51:662–64.

Jolly P. 2005. Medical school tuition and young physicians' indebtedness. Health Affairs 24(2):527–35.

Jones RF, Korn D. 1997. On the cost of educating a medical student. Academic Medicine 72(3):200–210.

Jordan RE, Wagner CL, Mascelli M, et al. 1996. Preclinical development of c7E3 Fab; a mouse/human chimeric monoclonal antibody fragment that inhibits platelet function by blockade of GPIIb/IIIa receptors with observations on the immunogenicity of c7E3 Fab in humans. In Horton MA, MD, ed., Adhesion Receptors as Therapeutic Targets. Boca Raton: CRC Press. 281–305.

Jovic E, Wallace JE, Lemaire J. 2006. The generation and gender shifts in medicine: an exploratory survey of internal medicine physicians. BMC Health Services Research 6:55–64.

Kan YW, Golbus MS, Trecartin R. 1975. Prenatal diagnosis of homozygous beta-thalassaemia. Lancet 2:790–91.

Kaplan SH, Sullivan LM, Dukes KA, et al. 1996. Sex differences in academic advancement. N. Engl. J. Med. 335:1283–89.

Kaushansky K. 1995. Thrombopoietin: the primary regulator of platelet production. Blood 86(2):419–31.

Kazazian HH Jr., Orkin SH, Markham AF, Chapman CR, Youssoufian H, Waber PG. 1984. Quantification of the close association between DNA haplotypes and specific beta-thalassaemia mutations in the Mediterraneans. Nature 310:152–54.

Kelley W, Randolph M, eds. 1994. *Careers in Clinical Research: Obstacles and Opportunities.* Washington, DC: National Academies Press.

Kennedy MM. 2003. Managing different generations requires new skills, insightful leadership. Physician Executive November–December:20–23

Keyser D, Lakoski JM, Lara-Cinisomo S, Schultz DJ, Williams VL, Zellers DF, Pincus HA. 2008. Advancing institutional efforts to support research mentorship: a conceptual framework and self-assessment tool. Acad. Med. 83:217–25.

Kirch DG, Salsberg E. 2007. The physician workforce challenge: response of the academic community. Ann. Surg. 246:535–40.

Komaromy M, Bindman AB, Haber RJ, Sande MA. 1993. Sexual harassment in medical training. N. Engl. J. Med. 328:322–26.

Korn D. 1998. Academic medical centers: whence they came, where they went. Journal of the Society for Gynecological Investigation 5(5):227–36.

Korn D. 2000. Conflicts of interest in biomedical research. JAMA 284(17):2234–37.

Korn D, Rich RR, Garrison H, et al. 2002. The NIH budget in the "post-doubling" era. Science 296(5572):1401–2.

Korn D, Stanski D, eds. 2006. Association of American Medical Colleges and the U.S. Food and Drug Administration. *Drug Development Science: Obstacles and Opportunities for Collaboration Among Academia, Industry, and Government.* Report of an invitational conference. Washington, DC: AAMC.

Korschun HW, Redding D, Teal GL, Johns MM. 2007. Realizing the vision of leadership development in an academic health center: the Woodruff Leadership Academy. Acad. Med. 82:264–71.

Kotchen TA, Lindquist T, Malik K, Ehrenfeld E. 2004. NIH peer review of grant applications for research. JAMA 291(7):836–43.

Kotchen TA, Lindquist T, Miller Sostek A, Hoffman R, Malik K, Stanfield B. 2006. Outcomes of National Institutes of Health peer review of clinical grant applications. Journal of Investigative Medicine 54:13–19.

Kralovec P, Miller JA, Wellikson L, Huddleston JM. 2006. The status of hospital medicine groups in the United States. J. Hosp. Med. 1:75–80.

Lambert EM, Holmboe ES. 2005. The relationship between specialty choice and gender of US medical students, 1990–2003. Acad. Med. 80(9):797–802.

Leboy P. 2008. Fixing the leaky pipeline: why aren't there many women in the top spots in academia? thescientist.com 22:67.

Lettre G, Sankaran VG, Bezerra MA, et al. 2008. DNA polymorphisms at the BCL11A, HBS1L-MYB, and beta-globin loci associate with fetal hemoglobin levels and pain crises in sickle cell disease. Proc Natl. Acad. Sci. USA 105:11869–74.

Levinson W, Kaufman K, Clark B, Tolle SW. 1991. Mentors and role models for women in academic medicine. West. J. Med. 154:423–26.

Lewis S. 1925. *Arrowsmith.* New York, Harcourt, Brace & Co.

Ley TJ, Hamilton BH. 2008. The gender gap in NIH grant applications. Science 322: 1472–74.

Ley TJ, Rosenberg L. 2002. Removing career obstacles for young physician-scientists: loan repayment programs. N. Engl. J. Med. 346:368–72.

Ley TJ, Rosenberg LE. 2005. The physician-scientist career pipeline in 2005: build it and they will come. JAMA 294(11):1343–51.

Lin YG. 1999. Bridging the worlds of medicine and science: an interview with Bert I. Shapiro, MD. JAMA 281:98–99.

Lopez MH, Marcelo KB. Fact Sheet, Center for Information and Research on Civic Learning and Engagement. 2006. Available at http://www.civicyouth.org/PopUps/youthdemo_2006.pdf, accessed June 30, 2008.

Loukopoulos D, Kaltysoya-Tassiopoulou A, Fessas P. 1988. Thalassemia control in Greece. Orig. Artic. Ser. Birth Defects 23:405–16.

Lovejoy FH Jr. 2004. Introduction of David G. Nathan and the 2003 John Howland Award. Pediatr. Res. 56:167–68.

Lucas AR. 1955. The influence of Leonardo da Vinci on the development of modern anatomy and physiology. Med. Bull. Ann Arbor 21:323–29.

Ludmerer KM. 1999. *Time to Heal: American Medical Education from the Turn of the Century to the Era of Managed Care.* New York: Oxford University Press.

Mallon WT, Bunton SA. 2005. *Characteristics of Research Centers and Institutes at US Medical Schools and Universities.* Washington, DC: AAMC.

Mark S, Link H, Morahan P, et al. 2001. Innovative mentoring programs to promote gender equity in academic medicine. Acad. Med. 76:39–42.

Marks AR. 2007. Physician-scientist, heal thyself....J. Clin. Invest. 117:2.

Martin MR, Lindquist T, Kotchen TA. 2008. Why are peer review outcomes less favorable for clinical science than for basic science grant applications? Am J Med. 121(7):637–41.

Martinez ED, Botos J, Dohoney KM, Geiman TM, Kolla SS, Olivera A, Qiu Y, Rayasam GV, Stavreva DA, Cohen-Fix O. 2007. Falling off the academic bandwagon. EMBO Reports 8:977–81.

McCarty M. 1985. *The Transforming Principle: Discovering That Genes Are Made of DNA.* New York: W. W. Norton & Company.

Melhado EM. 1999. Innovation and public accountability in clinical research. Millbank Quarterly 77:111–72.

Members of the First and Second Committees on Women Faculty in the School of Science. 1999. *A Study on the Status of Women Faculty in Science at MIT.* Cambridge: MIT Faculty Newsletter, March. Available at http://web.mit.edu/fnl/women.html, accessed Dec. 18, 2007.

Miles SM. 2005. *The Hippocratic Oath and the Ethics of Medicine.* New York: Oxford University Press.

Milner J, Hoffhines A. 2007. The discovery of aspirin's antithrombotic effects. Tex. Heart Inst. J. 34:179–86.

Mohan-Ram V. 2000. 'I Swear...': an oath for scientists and engineers. Science Careers (from the journal Science) 2000–11–10.

Morahan PS, Voytko ML, Abbuhl S, et al. 2001. Ensuring the success of women faculty at AMCs: lessons learned form the National Centers of Excellence in Women's Health. Acad. Med. 76(1):19–31.

Morzinski J, Simpson D, Bower D, Diehr S. 1994. Faculty development through formal mentoring. Acad. Med. 69:267–69.

Moss J, Teshima J, Leszcz M. 2008. Peer group mentoring for junior faculty. Acad. Psychiatry 32:230–35.

Nabel EG. 2008. *Issues Faced by Government Entities in Supporting the Physician-Scientist Workforce.* Association of Professors of Medicine Physician-Scientist Initiative: Recommendations for Revitalizing the Nation's Physician-Scientist Workforce. Available at http://dev.im.org/PolicyandAdvocacy/PolicyIssues/Research/PSI/Documents/APM%20PSI%20Report.pdf.pdf.

Nathan DG. 1974 Fetal research: an investigator's view. Villanova Law Rev. 22: 384–94.

Nathan DG. 1995. *Genes, Blood, and Courage: A Boy Called Immortal Sword.* Cambridge: Harvard University Press.

Nathan DG. 1998. Clinical research: perceptions, reality, and proposed solutions. JAMA 280:1427–31.

Nathan DG. 2002 Educational-debt relief for clinical investigators: a vote of confidence. N. Engl J. Med. 346:372–74.

Nathan DG. 2004. Acceptance of the 2003 John Howland Award: a journey in clinical research. Pediatr. Res. 56:169–76.

Nathan DG. 2005. The Several C's of Clinical Research. J. Clin. Invest. 115:795–97.

Nathan DG. 2007a. *The Cancer Treatment Revolution.* Hoboken, NJ: John Wiley and Sons.

Nathan DG. 2007b. Acceptance of the 2006 Kober Medal. J. Clin. Invest. 117:1107–13.

Nathan DG, Wilson JD. 2003. Clinical research and the NIH: a report card. N. Engl. J. Med. 349:1860–65.

National Academy of Sciences, National Academy of Engineering, and Institute of Medicine, Committee on Maximizing the Potential of Women in Academic Science and Engineering. 2006. *Beyond Bias and Barriers: Fulfilling the Potential of Women in Academic Science and Engineering.* Washington, DC: National Academies Press.

National Institutes of Health. 2008a. *Women in Research: The Involvement of Women in NIH Extramural Research, Training, and Career Development Programs.* Available at http://grants.nih.gov/grants/award/Research_Training_Investment/WOMEN_IN_RESEARCH_2.ppt, accessed March 10, 2008.

National Institutes of Health, Office of Extramural Research. 2008b. Average Age of Principal Investigators. NIH Extramural Data Book (electronic publication). Available at http://report.nih.gov/NIH_Investment/PDF_sectionwise/NIH_Extramural_DataBook_PDF/NEDB_SPECIAL_TOPIC-AVERAGE_AGE.pdf, accessed Oct. 23, 2008.

National Research Council of the National Academies. 2005. *Bridges to Independence: Fostering the Independence of New Investigators in Biomedical Research.* Washington, DC: National Academies Press.

Nelson B. 2007. Tips and techniques to bridge the generation gaps. Healthcare Registration January:3–5.

Nickerson KG, Bennett NM, Estes D, Shea S. 1990. The status of women at one academic medical center: breaking through the glass ceiling. JAMA 264(14):1813–17.

Noble D. 2006. *The Music of Life: Biology beyond the Genome.* Oxford: Oxford University Press.

Nonnemaker L. 2000. Women physicians in academic medicine: new insights from cohort studies. N. Engl. J. Med. 342:399–405.

Nuland SB. 2003. *The Doctors' Plague.* New York: W. W. Norton & Company.

Okin SM. 1989. *Justice, Gender, and the Family.* New York: Basic Books.

Palepu A, Friedman RH, Barnett RC, Carr PL, Ash AS, Szalacha L, Moskowitz MA. 1998. Junior faculty members' mentoring relationships and their professional development in US medical schools. Acad. Med. 73(3):318–23.

Pauling L, Itano H, Singer SJ, Wells I. 1949. Sickle cell anemia, a molecular disease. Science 110:543–48.

Pololi L, Knight S. 2005. Mentoring faculty in academic medicine. A new paradigm? J. Gen. Intern. Med. 20(9):866–70.

Pololi L, Knight S, Dennis K, Frankel R. 2002. Helping medical school faculty realize their dreams: an innovative, collaborative mentoring program. Acad. Med. 77:377–84.

Porter R. 1997. *The Greatest Benefit to Mankind: A Medical History of Humanity.* New York: W. W. Norton & Company.

Prensky M. 2005–6. Listen to the natives. Educational Leadership 63:8–13.

Raines C. 2003. *Connecting Generations: The Sourcebook for a New Workplace.* Menlo Park, Calif.: Crisp Publications.

Ramanan RA, Phillips RS, Davis RB, Silen W, Reede JY. 2002. Mentoring in medicine: keys to satisfaction. Am. J. Med. 112(4):336–41.

Rangel SJ, Efron B, Moss RL. 2002. Recent trends in National Institutes of Health funding of surgical research. Ann. Surg. 236(3):277–86.

Reese DM. 1998. Fundamentals: Rudolf Virchow and modern medicine. West. J. Med. 169:105–8.

Reich MH. 1986. The mentor connection. Personnel 63:50–56.

Rivera JA, Levine RB, Wright SM. 2005. Completing a scholarly project during residency training: perspectives of residents who have been successful. J. Gen. Intern. Med. 20(4):366–69.

Rivkees SA, Genel M. 2007. American pediatric academia: the looming question. J Pediatr. 151(3):223–24.

Robinson GC. 1957. *The Hospital of the Rockefeller Institute, 1910–1913. In Canby GC, ed., Adventures in Medical Education.* Cambridge: Commonwealth Fund, Harvard University Press. 81–100.

Roche GR. 1979. Much ado about mentors. Harvard. Bus. Rev. 1:14–28.

Rosenberg L. 1999. The physician-scientist: an essential—and fragile—link in the medical research chain. J. Clin. Invest. 103:1621–26.

Rotblat, Sir J. 1999. A Hippocratic Oath for scientists. Science. 286:1475.

Ryle, John. 1999 [1931]. The physician as scientist and naturalist. *Lancet* 354:1485.

Sambunjak D, Straus SE, Marušić A. 2006. Mentoring in academic medicine: a systematic review. JAMA 6:296(9):1103–15.

Schechter A. 1998. The crisis in clinical research. JAMA 280:1440–42.

Schubert C, Sinha G. 2004. A lab of her own. Nature Med. 10(2):114–15.

Seligsohn U, Mibashan RS, Rodeck CH, et al. 1985. Prenatal diagnosis of Glanzmann's thrombasthenia. Lancet 2:1419.

Sex/gender in the biomedical science workforce. 2005. Available at http://grants.nih.gov/grants/policy/sex_gender/q_a.htm, accessed April 17, 2008.

Shalev BA. 2005. *One Hundred Years of Nobel Prizes.* Los Angeles: Americas Group.

Shannon JA. 1987. The National Institutes of Health: some critical years, 1955–1957. Science 237:865–69.

Shields MC, Shields MT. 2003. Working with Generation X physicians. Physician Executive November–December:14–18.

Shulman LE. 1996. Clinical research, 1996: stirrings from the academic health centers. Academic Medicine 71(4):362–63.

Simmons JG. 2002. *Doctors and Discoveries: Lives That Created Today's Medicine.* Boston: Houghton Mifflin Company.

Sirridge MS. 1985. The mentor system in medicine: how it works for women. J. Am. Med. Womens Assoc. 2:51–53.

Skinner CA. 2006. Reinventing medical work and training: a view from Generation X. MJA 185:35–36.

Smith JW, Steinhubl SR, Lincoff AM, et al. 1999. Rapid platelet-function assay (RPFA): an automated and quantitative cartridge-based method. Circulation 99:620–25.

Smith LG. 2005. Medical professionalism and the generation gap. Am. J. Med. 118:439–42.

Souba WW. 2004. New ways of understanding and accomplishing leadership in academic medicine. J. Surg. Res. 117:177–86.

SPUSA Pledge. 2008. Student Pugwash USA. Available at http://www.spusa.org/pledge/, accessed March 26, 2009.

Starr P. 1982. *The Social Transformation of American Medicine.* New York: Basic Books.

Stokes DE. 1997. *Pasteur's Quadrant: Basic Science and Technological Innovation.* Washington, DC: Brookings Institution Press.

Stratton TD, McLaughlin MA, Witte FM, et al. 2005. Does students' exposure to gender discrimination and sexual harassment in medical school affect specialty choice and residency program selection? Acad. Med. 80:400–408.

Sung NS, Crowley WF Jr, Genel M, et al. 2003. Central challenges facing the national clinical research enterprise. JAMA 289:1278–87.

Tesch BJ, Wood HM, Helwig AL, Nattinger AB. 1995. Promotion of women physicians in academic medicine: glass ceiling or sticky floor? JAMA 273:1022–25.

Thomas CP, Conrad P, Casler R, Goodman E. 2006. Trends in the use of psychotropic medications among adolescents, 1994 to 2001. Psychiatr. Serv. 57:63–69.

Thompson JN, Moskowitz J. 1997. Preventing the extinction of the clinical research ecosystem. JAMA 278(3):241–45.

Tracy E, Jagsi R, Starr R, Tarbell NJ. 2004. Outcomes of a pilot faculty mentoring program. Am. J. Obstet. Gynecol. 191(6):1846–50.

Trower CA. 2007. Making academic dentistry more attractive to new teachers-scholars. J. Dental Ed. 71:601–5.

Trumble, W., and Brown L., eds. 2002. *Shorter Oxford English Dictionary.* Fifth ed. Oxford: Oxford University Press.

Tsai DF, Chen DS. 2003. An oath for bioscientists. J. Biomed. Sci. 10:569–76.

Ullman A. 2007. Pasteur-Koch: distinctive ways of thinking about infectious diseases. Microbe 2:383–87.

Ung NS, Crowley WF, Genel M, et al. 2003. Central challenges facing the national clinical research enterprise. JAMA 289(10):1278–87.

University of Kentucky. 2008. Physician Scientist Program Overview. Available at http://www.mc.uky.edu/medicine/administration/PSP.asp, accessed Jan. 12, 2009.

Varki A, Rosenberg LE. 2002. Emerging opportunities and career paths for the young physician-scientist. Nat. Med. 8(5):437–39.

Vesalius A. 1543. *De Humani Corporis Fabrica.* Basel: Oporini.

Waisbren SE, Bowles H, Hasan T, et al. 2008. Gender differences in research grant applications and funding outcomes for medical school faculty. J. Women's Health 17(2):207–14.

Wasserstein AG, Quistberg DA, Shea JA. 2007. Mentoring at the University of Pennsylvania: results of a faculty survey. J. Gen. Intern. Med. 22(2):210–14.

Weinberg RA. 2006. A lost generation. Cell 126:9–10.

Weinert CR, Billings J, Ryan R, Ingbar DH. 2006. Academic and career development of pulmonary and critical care physician-scientists. American Journal of Respiratory and Critical Care Medicine 173:23–31.

Williams RL, Johnson SB, Greene SM, et al. 2008. Signposts along the NIH roadmap for reengineering clinical research: lessons from the Clinical Research Networks Initiative. Archives of Internal Medicine 168(17):1919–23.

Wingard DL, Garman KA, Reznik V. 2004. Facilitating faculty success: outcomes and cost benefit of the UCSD National Center of Leadership in Academic Medicine. Acad. Med. 79:S9–11.

Witte FM, Stratton TD, Nora LM. 2006. Stories from the field: students' descriptions of gender discrimination and sexual harassment during medical school. Acad. Med. 81(7):648–54.

Wood AJ. 2006. A proposal for radical changes in the drug-approval process. N. Engl. J. Med. 355:618–23.

Woolf SH. 2008. The meaning of translational research and why it matters. JAMA 299:211–13.

Wright SM, Kern DE, Kolodner K, Howard DM, Brancati FL. 1998. Attributes of excellent attending-physician role models. N. Engl. J. Med. 339:1986–93.

Wyngaarden JB. 1979. The clinical investigator as an endangered species. N. Engl. J. Med. 301(23):1254–59.

Wyngaarden JB. 1987. The National Institutes of Health in its centennial year. Science 237:869–75.

Yedidia MJ, Bickel J. 2001. Why aren't there more women leaders in academic medicine? The views of clinical department chairs. Acad. Med. 76(5):453–65.

Zemke R, Raines C, Filipczak B. 2000. *Generations at Work: Managing the Clash of Veterans, Boomers, Xers, and Nexters in Your Workplace.* New York: American Management Association (AMACOM).

Zemlo T, Garrison H, Partridge N, Ley T. 2000. The physician-scientist: career issues and challenges at the year 2000. FASEB J. 14:221–30.

Zerhouni EA. 2005. Translational and clinical science: times for a new vision. N. Engl. J. Med. 353:1621–23.

Contributors

James M. Anderson, MD, PhD, is Professor and Chair of the Department of Cell and Molecular Physiology, University of North Carolina at Chapel Hill School of Medicine. He was previously Professor of Medicine at Yale University School of Medicine, where he had also trained in internal medicine and hepatology. Dr. Anderson directs the Howard Hughes Medical Institute–funded Translational Med-into-Grad program for PhD students at the University of North Carolina.

Ann J. Brown, MD, MHS, is Associate Professor of Medicine and Associate Vice Dean for Faculty Development at Duke University School of Medicine. Dr. Brown is an endocrinologist with research interests in polycystic ovary syndrome and type 2 diabetes, as well as professional development for women faculty.

Barry S. Coller, MD, is the David Rockefeller Professor, Vice President for Medical Affairs, and Physician-in-Chief at Rockefeller University. He is also the Principal Investigator of the university's NIH-funded Clinical and Translational Science Award. Previously Chief of Hematology at the State University of New York at Stony Brook and Chair of the Department of Medicine at Mount Sinai School of Medicine, Dr. Coller is a member of the Institute of Medicine and the National Academy of Sciences, a former President of the American Society of Hematology, and President of the new Society for Clinical and Translational Science. He is engaged in translational research aimed at preventing and treating thrombosis and monitoring antiplatelet therapy.

Fabio Cominelli, MD, PhD, is the Hermann Menges, Jr Chair in Internal Medicine and Chief of the Division of Gastrointenstinal and Liver Disease at Case Western University. He is also Director of the Case Western Reserve University Digestive Health Center and the University Hospital Case Medical Center Digestive Health and Disease Service Line. Prior to these appointments in 2008, Dr. Cominelli was the David D. Stone Professor of Medicine and Chief of the Division of Gastroenterology and Hepatology at the University of Virginia. His research is in the area of cytokine networks and mucosal immunity.

Paul E. DiCorleto, PhD, is Chairman of both the Lerner Research Institute of the Cleveland Clinic and the Department of Molecular Medicine at Case Western Reserve University School of Medicine. He received his doctorate in biochemistry from Cornell University. Dr. DiCorleto's research focuses on the molecular and cellular basis of atherosclerosis.

Mark Donowitz, MD, is the LeBoff Professor for Research in Digestive Diseases, Professor of Medicine and Physiology, and Director of the Center for Epithelial Disorders at the Johns Hopkins School of Medicine. He held previous academic appointments at the New England Medical Center and the Tufts University School of Medicine. As President of the American Gastroenterological Association, Dr. Donowitz worked to combat physician-scientist dropout by initiating a bridging grants program for young scientists. His research interests are in molecular mechanisms of regulation of epitheal transport proteins and protein-protein interactions.

Stephen G. Emerson, MD, PhD, became the thirteenth President of Haverford College in 2007. He was previously the Francis C. Wood Professor of Medicine, Pathology, and Pediatrics, and Chief of the Division of Hematology-Oncology at the University of Pennsylvania. Prior to that he served on the faculties of the University of Michigan and Harvard Medical School. Dr. Emerson is a stem cell biologist.

Gregory Germino, MD, is Professor of Medicine, Molecular Biology, and Genetics at the Johns Hopkins University School of Medicine and an Affiliate Member of the McKusick-Nathans Institute of Genetic Medicine. An NIH MERIT awardee, former Councilor of the American Society for Clinical Investigation, and a member of the Board of Directors of FASEB, Dr. Germino's research interest is in defining the mechanisms that regulate renal tubular morphology.

Stephen J. Heinig is Lead Science Policy Analyst with the Association of American Medical Colleges. He joined the association in 1997 and served on the staff of the AAMC's two task forces on clinical research. Previously, Mr. Heinig was a Science Policy Analyst at FASEB.

Margaret K. Hostetter, MD, is the Jean McLean Wallace Professor and Chair of the Department of Pediatrics at Yale University School of Medicine. She received her MD from Baylor College of Medicine and did her postgraduate training at Boston Children's Hospital and Harvard Medical School. Her research focuses on microbial pathogenesis. Dr. Hostetter has led the NIH-funded Pediatric Scientist Development Program since 1996, is a past president of the Society for Pediatric Research, and is a member of the Institute of Medicine of the National Academy of Sciences.

Reshma Jagsi, MD, DPhil, is Assistant Professor of Radiation Oncology at the University of Michigan. A physician-researcher and social scientist trained at Harvard and Oxford Universities, she has conducted a number of studies investigating women's participation in academic medicine, barriers to their advancement, and interventions targeted to increase their representation. Dr. Jagsi's clinical research focuses on improving the quality of care received by patients with breast cancer.

Kenneth Kaushansky, MD, is the Helen M. Ranney Professor of Medicine and Chair of the Department of Medicine at the University of California, San Diego. He is past president of the American Society for Clinical Investigation and the American Society of Hematology, former editor-in-chief of *Blood,* and a member of the Institute of Medicine of the National Academy of Sciences. Dr. Kaushansky's translational research is in the fields of hematopoietic stem cells, megakaryopoiesis and thrombopoietin.

David Korn, MD, is the Vice Provost for Research at Harvard University and Professor of Pathology at Harvard Medical School. From 1997 to 2008 he served as Senior Vice President for Biomedical and Health Sciences Research and in 2008 as Chief Scientific Officer of the Association of American Medical Colleges in Washington, D.C. Previously he was the Carl and Elizabeth Naumann Professor and Dean of the Stanford University School of Medicine from 1984 to 1995 and Vice President of Stanford University from 1986 to 1995.

Timothy J. Ley, MD, is the Alan and Edith Wolff Professor of Medicine and Professor of Genetics at Washington University, St. Louis. Dr. Ley is past president of the American Society for Clinical Investigation, treasurer of the American Association of Physicians, fellow of the American Association for the Advancement of Science, and a member of the Institute of Medicine of the National Academy of Sciences. He has written extensively about the physician-scientist career path and was an advocate for establishing the extramural Loan Repayment Program at the National Institutes of Health.

Philip M. Meneely, PhD, is Professor of Biology at Haverford College where he previously served as Associate Provost and Chair of the Department of Biology. Professor Meneely received his PhD in Genetics from the University of Minnesota and conducts research on the genes that affect the process of meiosis. In addition, Dr. Meneely develops curriculum targeted toward training future biomedical researchers, such as his most recent book, *Advanced Genetic Analysis.*

David G. Nathan, MD, is President Emeritus of the Dana Farber Cancer Institute in Boston and the Robert A. Stranahan Distinguished Professor of Pediatrics and Professor of Medicine at Harvard Medical School. He is the former Chief of Hematology, Chairman of the Department of Pediatrics, and Physician-in-Chief of Children's Hospital, Boston, and the Harvard Medical School. Among his notable contributions were the elucidation of the pathophysiologic basis of thalassemia, the development of prenatal diagnostic testing, pioneering iron chelation therapy, the development of hydroxyurea therapy of sickle cell disease and major additions to our current understanding of hematopoiesis. Dr. Nathan served as Chairman of the NIH Director's Panel on Clinical Research, which between 1995 and 1997 developed groundbreaking recommendations to promote clinical research and clinical investigators. He has been the recipient of the National Medal of Science, the Howland Medal of the American Pediatric Society, the Henry Stratton Medal of the American Society of Hematology, and the Kober Medal of the Association of American Physicians.

Philip A. Pizzo, MD, became Dean of the Stanford University School of Medicine in 2001. Previously he was Physician-in-Chief of Children's Hospital, Boston, and Chair of the Department of Pediatrics at Harvard Medical School (1996-2001) and head of the Infectious Diseases Section and Chief of Pediatrics at the National Cancer Institute, where he also served as Acting Scientific Director before moving to Boston. Dr. Pizzo and his research team pioneered the development of new treatments for children with HIV infection, among other innovations in cancer and infectious diseases.

Jennifer Punt, VMD, PhD, is Professor of Biology at Haverford College. She is a graduate of the VMD-PhD program of the University of Pennsylvania. Dr. Punt, whose research is on negative selection in immune regulation, has trained a large number of undergraduate students in biomedical research, many of whom have continued to graduate and medical schools at leading universities.

Andrew I. Schafer, MD, is the E. Hugh Luckey Distinguished Professor of Medicine and Chair of the Department of Medicine at Weill Cornell Medical College and Physician-in-Chief of the New York–Presbyterian Hospital–Weill Cornell Medical Center. His prior positions were the Frank Thomas Wister Professor and Chair of the Department of Medicine at the University of Pennsylvania School of Medicine, Chair of the Department of Medicine at Baylor College of Medicine, Chief of Medicine at the Houston Veterans Affairs Medical Center, and ten years on the faculty of Harvard Medical School and the Brigham and Women's Hospital. An investigator in the area of thrombosis, platelet, and vascular cell biology, Dr. Schafer is past president of the American Society of Hematology and President-Elect of the Association of Professors of Medicine.

Alan L. Schwartz, MD, PhD, is the Harriet B. Spoehrer Professor of Pediatrics and Chairman of the Department of Pediatrics at Washington University School of Medicine, St. Louis. He has led the NIH-funded Child Health Research Center since 1994 and has directed the Markey Pathway in Human Pathobiology at Washington University since 1991. Dr. Schwartz's research focuses on receptor biology, protein trafficking, and turnover. He is a member of the Institute of Medicine of the National Academy of Sciences.

Roy L. Silverstein, MD, is Chair of the Department of Cell Biology, occupies the Jan Bleeksma Chair in Vascular Cell Biology and Atherosclerosis, and is Vice Chair of the Lerner Research Institute of the Cleveland Clinic. Prior to assuming his current positions in 2004, he was Chief of the Division of Hematology-Oncology at Weill Cornell Medical College. Dr. Silverstein's research focuses on the molecular and cellular basis of human vascular diseases. He is also active in medical and PhD education and in national advocacy for research and education.

Nancy J. Tarbell, MD, is the C.C. Wang Professor of Radiation Oncology at the Massachusetts General Hospital and in 2008 became Dean for Academic and Clinical Programs at Harvard Medical School. Dr. Tarbell is an international authority in pediatric radiation oncology with special expertise in pediatric neuro-oncology.

Index